# Physical Signs in Orthopaedics

# Physical Signs in Orthopaedics

## Henry John Walsh

**MB, ChB, MChOrth, FRCS(Eng)**
**Senior Lecturer**

## Leslie Klenerman

**ChM, FRCS(Eng), FRCS(Ed)**
**Professor**

Department of Orthopaedic and Accident Surgery
University of Liverpool

BMJ
Publishing
Group

First published in 1994
by the BMJ Publishing Group, BMA House, Tavistock Square,
London WC1H 9JR

**British Library Cataloguing in Publication Data**

A catalogue record for this book is available
from the British Library

ISBN 0-7279-0845-6

Typeset by Apek Typesetters Ltd, Nailsea, Bristol
Printed and bound in Great Britain at the University Press, Cambridge

# Contents

Introduction    vii

**1**  Shoulder and upper arm    1

**2**  Elbow and forearm    12

**3**  Hand and wrist    17

**4**  Axial skeleton    37

**5**  Hip and pelvis    44

**6**  Knee    50

**7**  Lower leg/tibia    59

**8**  Foot    65

**9**  Miscellaneous conditions    85

Index    91

# Introduction

In orthopaedics it is essential to recognise and evaluate clinical signs. To a large extent this is a result of practice and experience. However, evidence of pathology can be seen only if the possible variations of the normal and abnormal are known. The idea of producing this book is to help students and practitioners familiarise themselves with the more common physical signs and at the same time encourage careful observation of patients. The text is short but it is hoped that the reader will be stimulated to consult other books and to learn more about the fascinating subject of orthopaedics.

It is recommended that readers look at one chapter at a time and write down the answers before checking the correct answers at the back of the chapter.

It is not possible to collect suitable examples of physical signs without the help of colleagues and we are grateful to all who have kindly allowed us to copy interesting slides. It is invidious to name particular individuals so we shall confine ourselves to stating that this has been a team effort from orthopaedic surgeons and physicians in Liverpool. We would also like to thank the members of the Photographic Departments at the Children's Hospital, Alder Hey and the Royal Liverpool University Hospital for their expertise and patience.

**Henry John Walsh**
**Leslie Klenerman**

# 1 Shoulder and upper arm

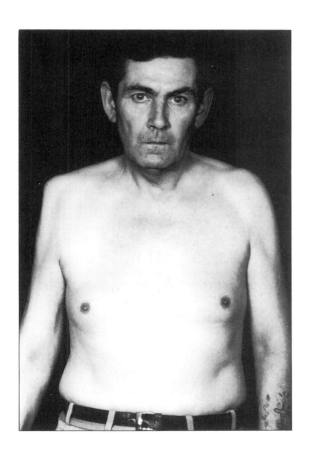

## 1.1

Six weeks before this photograph was taken this man fell and injured his right shoulder. He did not immediately seek medical advice but was referred to the hospital because his shoulder was still stiff and uncomfortable.

> **What injury has he sustained?**

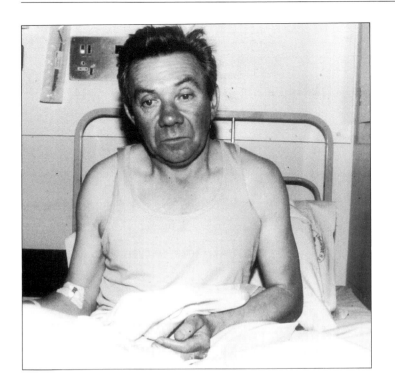

## 1.2 and 1.3

This man fell and injured his left shoulder. The photograph was taken when the doctor asked him to externally rotate his shoulders. He has good movement on the right side but, as you can see, he has restricted movement on the left.

> What is the clinical diagnosis?
>
> How would you confirm this radiologically?

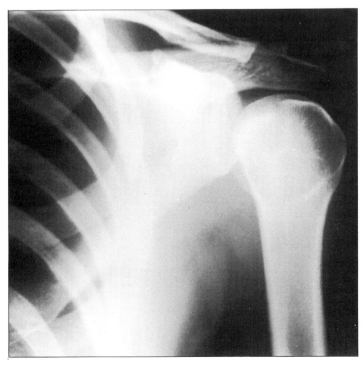

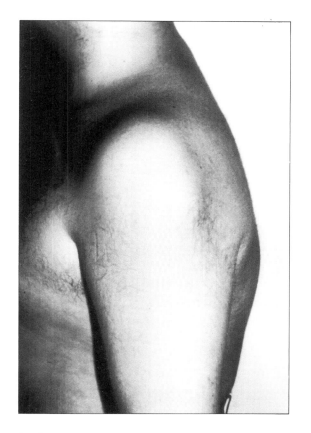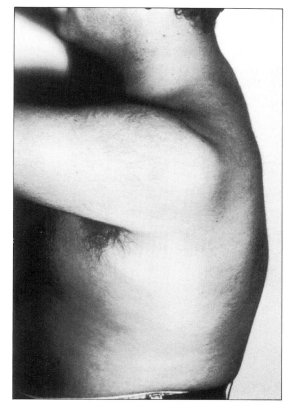

# 1.4 and 1.5

The range of movement in this young man's left shoulder is excessive, and he can control it at will. By a trick movement he is able to manipulate his humerus posteriorly as shown in the photograph.

---

**What condition does he have?**

---

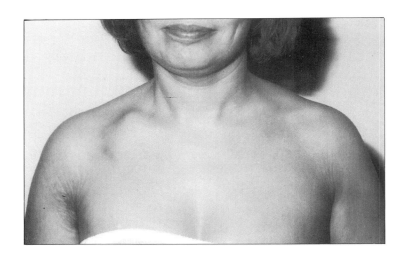

## 1.6

This woman had sustained an injury to her right arm 9 months before this photograph was taken, when she fell onto her outstretched right hand.

---

What injury has she sustained?

What has been the outcome?

---

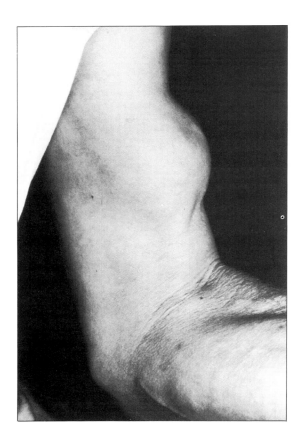

## 1.7

This middle aged man experienced spontaneous pain on the anterior aspect of both upper arms. He then noticed swellings developing, particularly when he flexed his elbows.

---

What is the diagnosis?

---

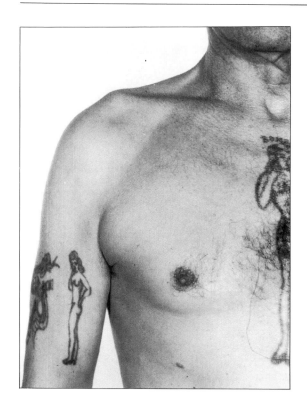

## **1.8** and **1.9**

The region of the right shoulder in this man, who was a keen rugby player, has become increasingly painful.

---
**What is the diagnosis?**
---

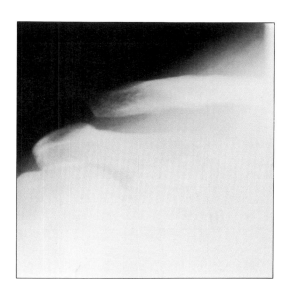

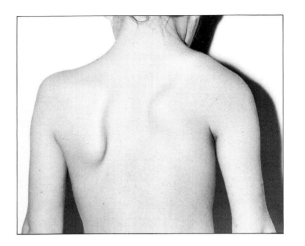

# 1.10

The girl in this photograph was born with a deformity of her right shoulder. As a consequence she has limited movement of the shoulder girdle.

> **What is the cause of this deformity?**

# 1.11

> **Describe the anomaly in this 8 year old boy.**

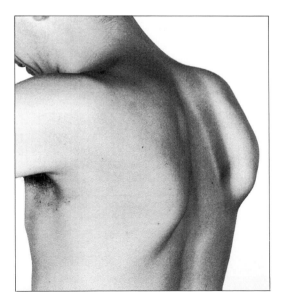

# 1.12

After recovering from a febrile illness a young man noticed that he had a problem with his right shoulder. This photograph shows the patient pushing against a wall with his hands and a deformity developing in his right shoulder girdle.

> **Describe the deformity.**
>
> **What is the cause?**

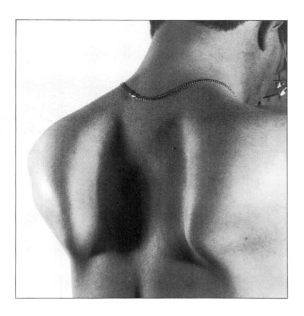 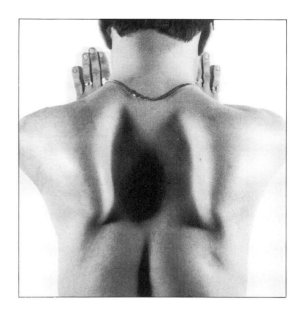

## 1.13 and 1.14

The young man in these photographs has a muscle disorder and, like the previous patient, shows deformity of his shoulder girdle when he presses against a wall. This deformity involves both scapulas. He also has some facial weakness.

What is the diagnosis?

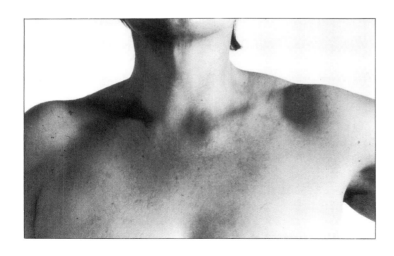

## 1.15

The area over the left sternoclavicular joint of this woman became painful, the joint became swollen and warm and was very tender to the touch. She was generally unwell with a high temperature.

What is the diagnosis?

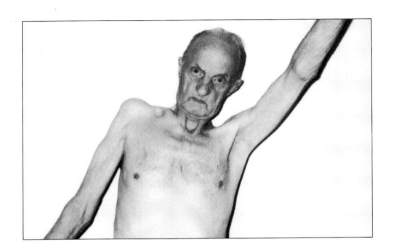

## 1.16

This elderly man sustained a dislocation of his right shoulder. Following the injury he was unable to abduct his right shoulder, as shown in this photograph.

> **What is your differential diagnosis?**

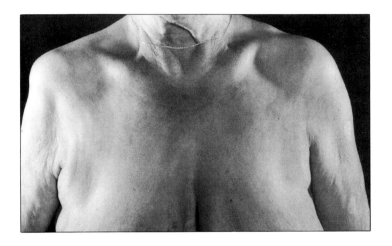

## 1.17 and 1.18

These photographs were taken 3 months after this elderly woman dislocated her right shoulder.

> **What physical sign does she exhibit?**

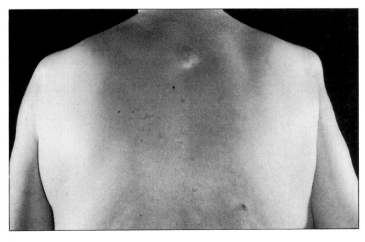

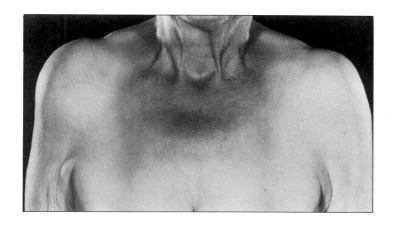

## 1.19

This patient has a generalised joint disorder and presented with a swelling in the region of the right shoulder.

> **What is the cause of the swelling?**

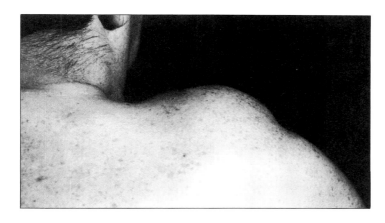

## 1.20

There is a fleshy swelling over the superior aspect of the shoulder girdle of this man. It does not transilluminate and is painless.

> **What could this swelling be?**

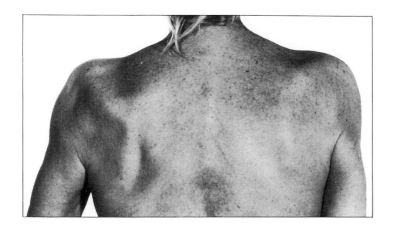

## 1.21

This young woman has pain in her left shoulder following an injury that she sustained some months before.

> **What physical signs does she exhibit?**

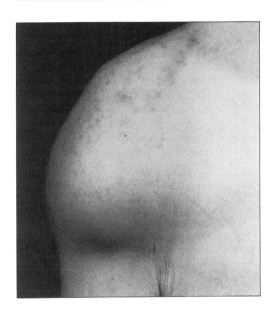

## 1.22

A swelling of the right shoulder joint, involving the anterior and lateral aspect of the upper arm, is visible in this patient.

> **What is the possible diagnosis?**

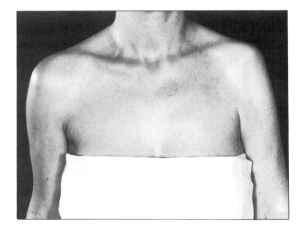

## 1.23

This woman has a generalised joint disorder, which also affects her left shoulder.

> **What do you think is the underlying condition?**

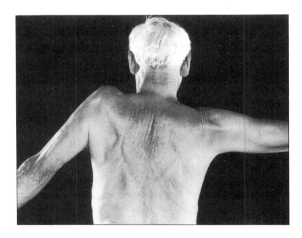

## 1.24

This man has been asked to abduct his shoulders. He is having problems on the left side.

> **What physical signs does he exhibit?**

# Answers to Chapter 1

**1.1**    Anterior dislocation of the right shoulder. Note the flattening of the normal shoulder contour and slight fullness in the deltopectoral region below the clavicle. Ninety per cent of shoulders dislocate anteriorly.

**1.2** and **1.3**    Posterior dislocation of the left shoulder. An anteroposterior radiograph will show the classic drumstick appearance of the upper humerus. If there is still doubt an axillary view will confirm the diagnosis.

**1.4** and **1.5**    Habitual posterior dislocation of the shoulder.

**1.6**    Fracture of the middle third of the clavicle, the outcome being malunion of the fracture.

**1.7**    Spontaneous rupture of the long head of biceps.

**1.8** and **1.9**    Dislocation of the right acromioclavicular joint. The diagnosis is confirmed on a radiograph comparing the right and left sides.

**1.10**    Sprengel's shoulder. This is a congenital anomaly associated with a small fixed scapula. It causes deformity of the shoulder girdle and decreases the range of motion.

**1.11**    Congenital amputation (terminal transverse) of the humerus. This condition is also known as phocomelia.

**1.12**    Winging of the right scapula. This deformity is sometimes associated with a viral infection, or injury leading to a palsy of the long thoracic nerve (neuralgic amyotrophy).

**1.13** and **1.14**    Winged scapulae associated with facioscapulo humeral dystrophy.

**1.15**    Septic arthritis of the sternoclavicular joint.

**1.16**    (a) Axillary nerve palsy.
(b) Complete rupture of the rotator cuff.

**1.17** and **1.18**    Wasting of the deltoid, giving a squared off shoulder contour due to an axillary nerve palsy.

**1.19**    Subacromial bursitis associated with rheumatoid arthritis.

**1.20**    A subcutaneous lipoma.

**1.21**    Wasting of the deltoid and spinati muscles following a dislocation on the left side.

**1.22**    The patient has a subdeltoid bursa.

**1.23**    Rheumatoid arthritis, leading to secondary arthritis of the left shoulder associated with a high riding humerus and wasting of the musculature.

**1.24**    The shrugging sign associated with a rupture of the rotator cuff, giving rise to decreased active abduction of the shoulder.

# 2  Elbow and forearm

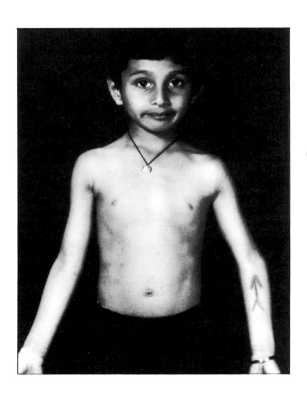

## 2.1

This 10 year old boy sustained an injury to his left elbow 4 years before this photograph was taken.

> **How would you describe the deformity?**

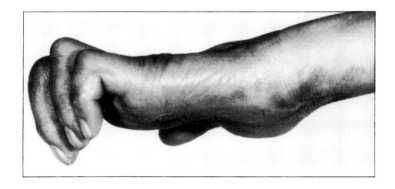

## 2.2

This patient had a supracondylar fracture as a child. Subsequently severe pain developed in the forearm, and stiffness and loss of function of the hand gradually increased.

> **How would you describe this fixed deformity?**

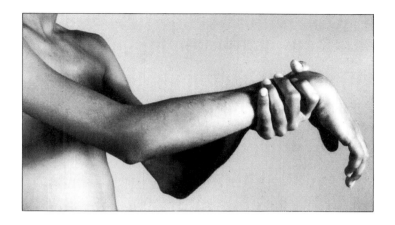

## 2.3

A fracture of the lower part of the humerus of this young man was treated conservatively. The day after the injury the patient was noted to have some weakness of his hand and wrist. This photograph shows the problem he encounters when he tries to extend his wrist and fingers.

Describe the deformity.

What is the cause of his lack of function?

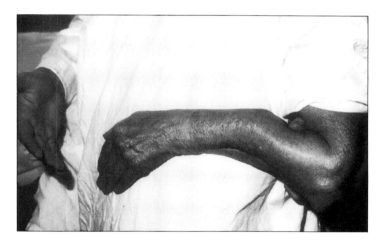

## 2.4 and 2.5

This elderly woman sustained an injury to her forearm 18 months before these photographs were taken. The deformity of the forearm is correctable, as shown in these photographs. She experiences no pain when her forearm is moved.

What is the reason for the mobility?

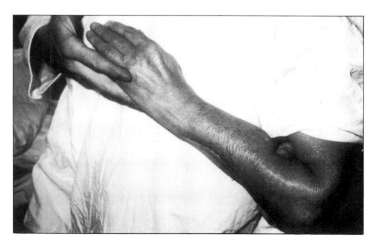

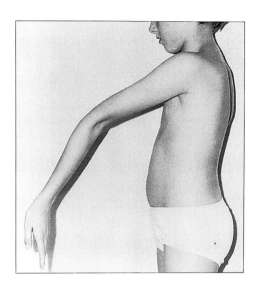

## 2.6

This 7 year old boy exhibits the physical signs shown in the photograph when his elbows are extended.

> **What is the reason for this?**
>
> **Which other areas of the body exhibit this phenomenon?**

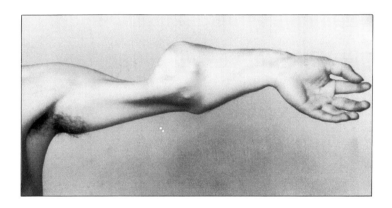

## 2.7

This young man has an inherited disorder affecting his skeleton. It has left him with deformity of the arm. He has other, asymptomatic, lesions in various other bones of his body.

> **What underlying disorder does he suffer from?**

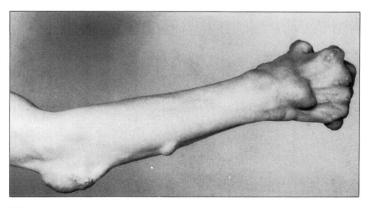

## 2.8

The photograph shows the forearm, elbow, and wrist of a middle aged man with a generalised joint disorder. Fleshy, subcutaneous lumps are visible along the extensor aspect of his arm.

> **What might these be?**

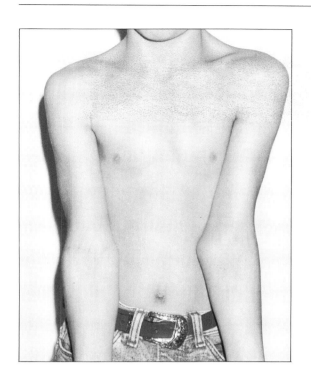

## 2.9

This young man has had an injury to his left elbow in the past and has developed deformity at this site.

| How would you describe this? |
| --- |

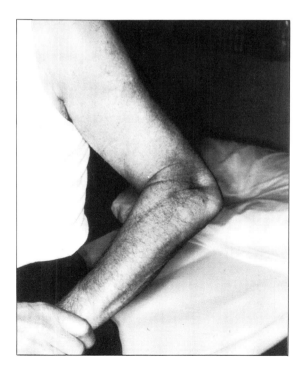

## 2.10

This man fell on to his outstretched left hand and injured his left elbow.

| What injury has he sustained? |
| --- |

## Answers to Chapter 2

**2.1**   Cubitus varus. This deformity does not affect function but this boy was about to undergo correction by supracondylar osteotomy for cosmetic reasons.

**2.2**   This is Volkmann's ischaemic contracture. It is the end result of an untreated compartment syndrome, is preventable—and when it occurs it is a disaster.

**2.3**   Drop wrist., which is caused by a complete radial nerve palsy.

**2.4** and   A fracture of the radius and ulna has gone on to non-union and the patient has developed a
**2.5**   pseudoarthrosis of the bones involved.

**2.6**   Hypermobility of the joints, showing hyperextension at the elbow. Hyperextension may also be found in the knees and hyperdorsiflexion in the metacarpophalangeal joints of the fingers.

**2.7**   Diaphysial aclasis or hereditary multiple exostoses.

**2.8**   Rheumatoid nodules. These are of prognostic significance and associated with more aggressive forms of the disease.

**2.9**   Cubitus valgus. If untreated this deformity will result in ulnar neuritis.

**2.10**   A posterior dislocation of the elbow.

# 3 Hand and wrist

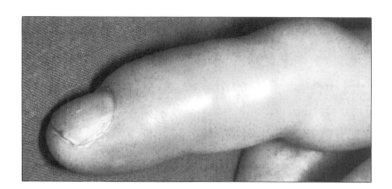

## Infection

### 3.1

This patient developed a swollen, red and painful index finger a few days after working in the garden.

> **What is your diagnosis?**

### 3.2

This patient had pricked his finger on a rose thorn many months before this picture was taken.

> **What is the lesion called?**
>
> **Why does it persist?**

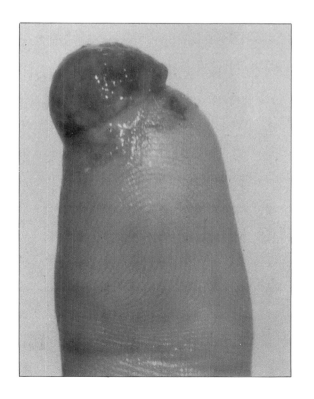

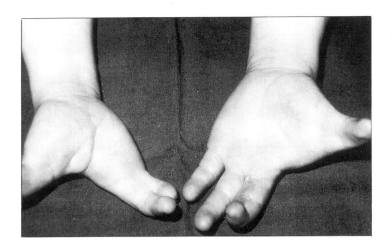

# Congenital

## 3.3

The patient in this photograph was born with these hand anomalies.

> **What are they called?**

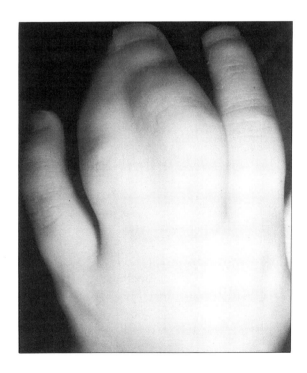

## 3.4

> **What is the name of this congenital anomaly of the hand?**
>
> **What is the accepted treatment?**

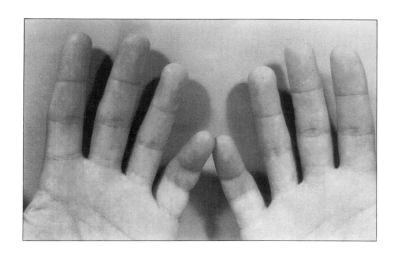

## 3.5 and 3.6

The little fingers of this young girl were bent, but caused no particular problems.

| What is the congenital abnormality? |
| --- |

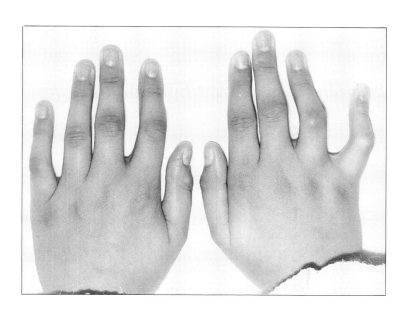

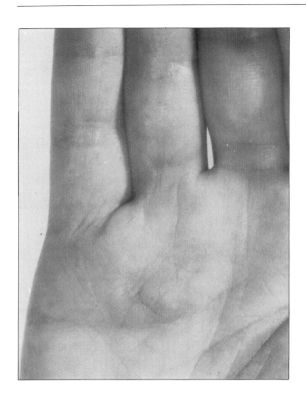

## **3.7** and **3.8**

This man noticed a thickening in the palm of his hand at the base of his ring finger. This was associated with a small pit. He also has fleshy swellings over the dorsal aspects of his proximal interphalangeal joints.

---

**What condition is he suffering from?**

---

**What are the lesions on the dorsum of the fingers?**

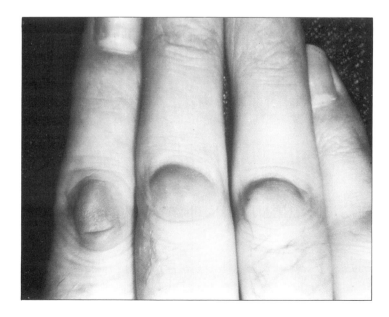

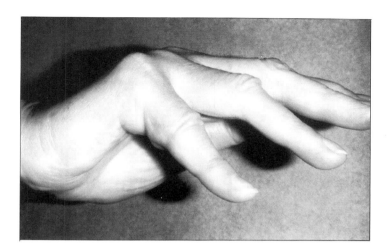

## **3.9** and **3.10**

Both of these patients have Dupuytren's disease and both are about to undergo surgery.

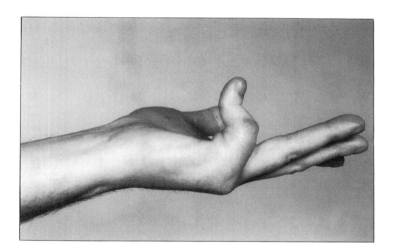

In which patient is fasciectomy more likely to be effective?

Where else would you look for this disease process?

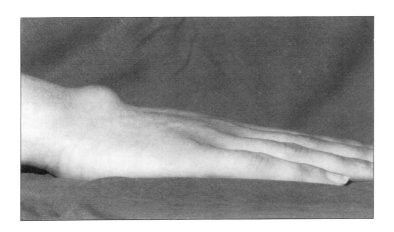

## Acquired

## 3.11

This young man developed a spontaneous swelling over the dorsum of his right wrist.

> **What is the lesion most likely to be?**

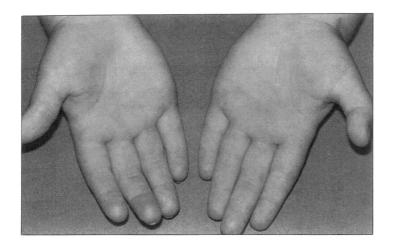

## 3.12

This woman experienced difficulties in extending her left thumb. When it did straighten it went back with a sudden 'click', which she felt at the volar aspect of her thumb. On examination there was some thickening over the region of the flexor tendons.

> **What condition does she have?**

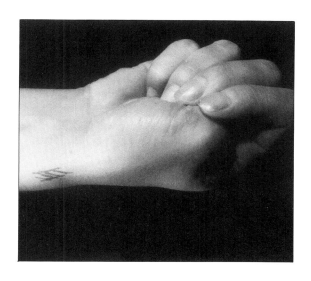

## 3.13

When this right handed woman squeezes her thumb into the palm of her hand, as shown in the photograph, she develops severe pain over the radial aspect of her wrist (as marked on her skin in the photograph). This pain increases if the wrist is passively moved into ulnar deviation. The patient also has pain over the area if she does any sustained activity with her hand, such as housework or racket sports.

---

**What condition does she suffer from?**

---

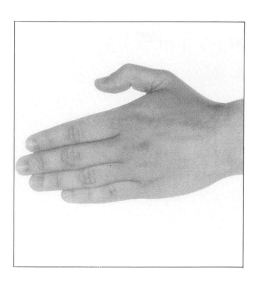

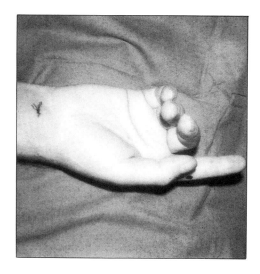

## 3.14

The patient fractured his left wrist 6 weeks ago. The fracture healed without problems, but after removal of the cast he was unable to straighten his left thumb.

---

**What problem has he developed?**

**Name three other recognised complications that follow distal radial fractures.**

---

## 3.15

This patient fell on to broken glass and cut his left wrist.

---

**Looking at the attitude of his hand, and the fingers, what structures has he almost certainly divided?**

---

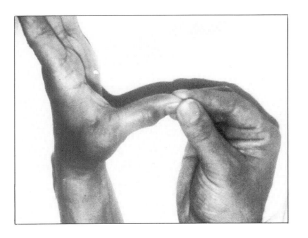
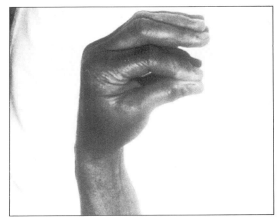

# 3.16, 3.17 and 3.18

Since this woman sustained an injury to her left thumb she has had problems with her pinch grip between the thumb and index finger. Her left thumb is more mobile than before the injury compared with the right thumb. This excess mobility is demonstrated in the photographs.

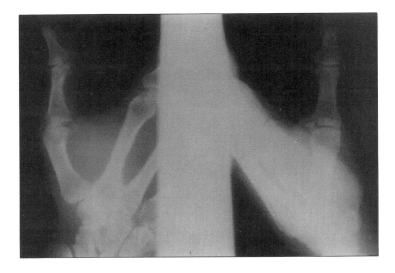

> What injury has she sustained?
>
> What is a common name for this problem in its chronic form?

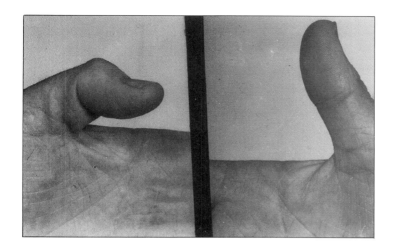

## 3.19

This man developed problems with his left thumb after being hit on the tip while trying to catch a cricket ball. He has been unable to straighten his thumb actively since the injury.

> **What structure has he damaged?**
>
> **What is the deformity commonly called?**

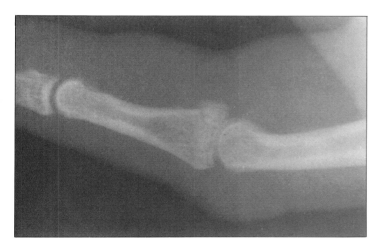

## 3.20

This is a radiograph of a patient with an extension injury to the right little finger. He did not initially seek medical advice, and subsequently developed the deformity shown in Photograph 3.21.

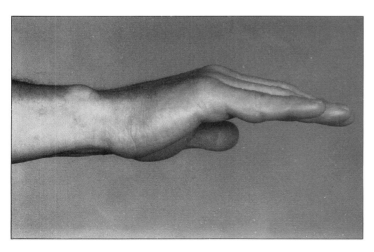

## 3.21

> **What injury has he sustained?**
>
> **Why has the deformity to his finger developed?**

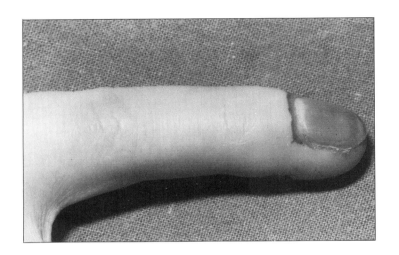

## 3.22

This patient trapped the tip of his finger in a car door.

> **What causes the blue dis-coloration under the nail?**
>
> **What injury is likely to be evident on a radiograph?**
>
> **How is this condition best treated by first aid?**

# Neurology

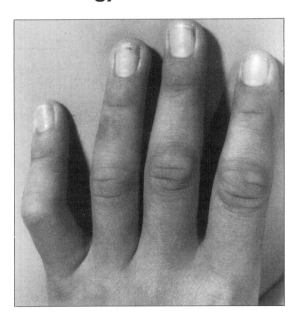

## 3.23

This woman complained of paraesthesia over the ring and little finger of her left hand on both the volar and dorsal aspects. She also noticed a deformity developing in the little finger.

> **What nerve lesion do you suspect?**

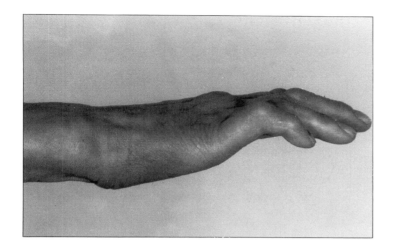

## 3.24

This patient has problems with his right hand involving the ring and little finger similar to those in the patient shown in Photograph 3.23.

> **How do the two deformities of the little finger differ, and how can you explain this difference neurologically?**

## 3.25 and 3.26

These photographs demonstrate a particular test for ulnar nerve function.

> **What is the test called, and what is the rationale behind it?**

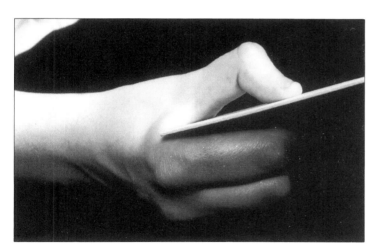

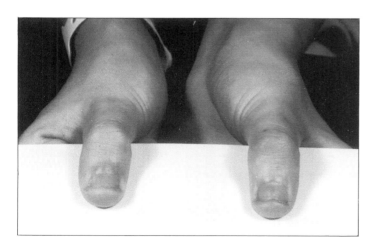

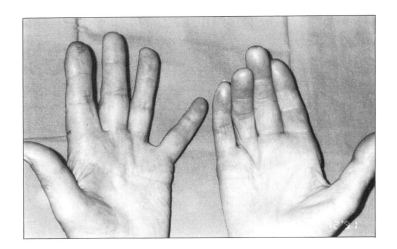

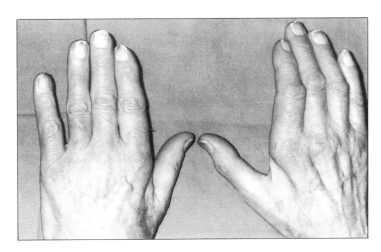

## 3.27 and 3.28

This patient has an ulnar nerve lesion affecting both hands, and demonstrates several physical signs.

> Describe three of these signs.

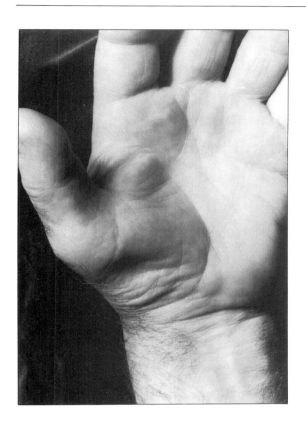

## 3.29

This patient suffered paraesthesia over the radial aspect of the hand, also involving the thumb and radial fingers, associated with pain in his hand and wrist which wakes him at night. The problem has continued for several months.

> **What physical sign does he demonstrate?**
>
> **Why does it develop?**

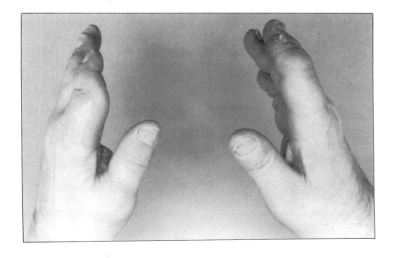

## 3.30

This patient has generalised arthritis, and a scaly skin condition with associated pitting of the nails of her fingers and thumb.

> **What is the underlying cause of the arthropathy?**

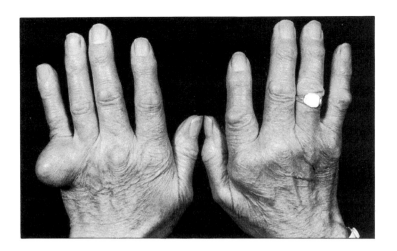

## 3.31

The swelling on this patient's left hand is solid and does not transilluminate. She has a generalised joint disease.

> **What might the lesion be?**

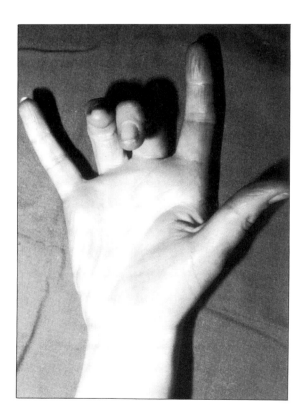

## 3.32

This patient has rheumatoid arthritis. She is unable to straighten the ring and middle fingers of her right hand without eliciting a click within the palm.

> **What problem has she developed?**
>
> **What is the underlying mechanism?**

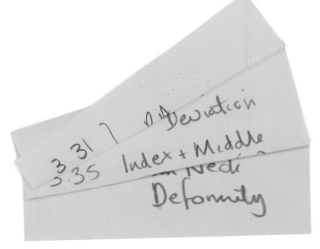

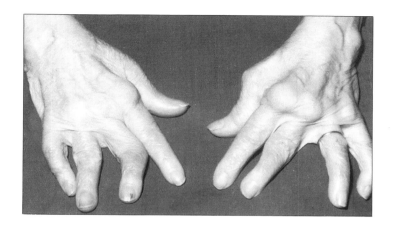

## 3.33

From what condition is this patient suffering?

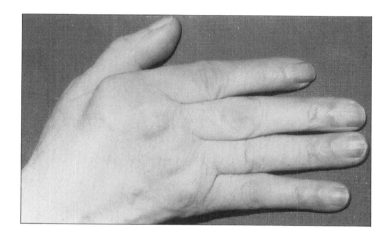

## 3.34

This patient suffers from the same condition as the patient in the previous photograph.

What is the classic deformity she exhibits at the metacarpophalangeal joint?

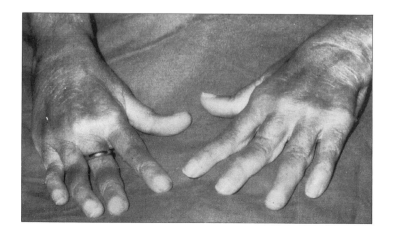

## 3.35

The patient shown here also suffers from the joint disorder described in Photographs 3.33 and 3.34.

Describe the deformity of the left index and middle fingers.

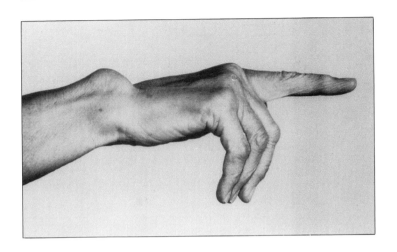

## 3.36

A patient developed severe synovitis involving many joints, particularly the dorsal aspect of his right wrist. As a consequence he noticed increasing problems with the medial three fingers of his right hand.

| What has happened? |
| --- |

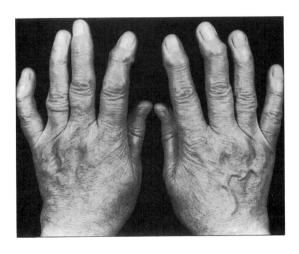 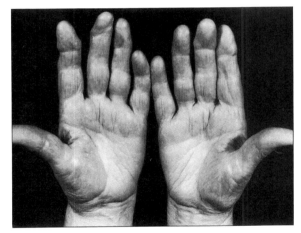

## 3.37 and 3.38

This woman has a family history of generalised osteoarthritis involving the large joints. She also has finger deformities, particularly of the distal interphalangeal joints of both hands.

| What are these nodules called? |
| --- |

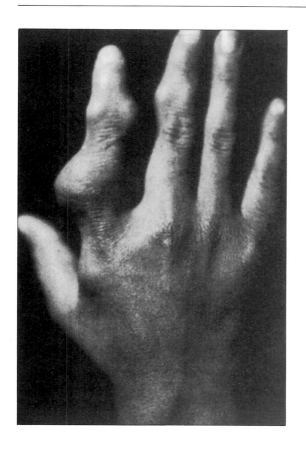

## 3.39

Here is a photograph of the index finger of an overweight 54 year old man who presented with pain in his great toe and effusion of his right knee joint. He later noted deformity and swelling of the distal interphalangeal joint of his index finger and erythema surrounded by tiny white nodules.

> **What form of arthropathy does he suffer from?**

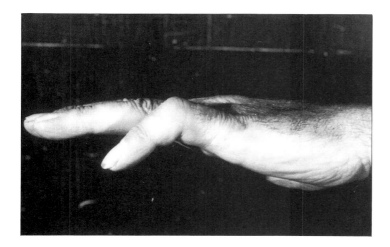

## 3.40

> **What structure has been severed as a result of a cut on the dorsal aspect of the proximal phalanx of this patient's little finger?**

# Answers to Chapter 3

## Infection

**3.1**      Acute suppurative tenosynovitis, which required urgent surgery.

**3.2**      Infected granuloma. Foreign material, probably part of the rose thorn in this particular case, has been retained in the wound.

## Congenital

**3.3**      Lobster hands. They are usually associated with similar deformities in the feet.

**3.4**      Syndactyly. An attempt should be made to separate the digits surgically, if possible.

**3.5** and **3.6**      Campodactyly (congenital flexion deformity of the digits). The little finger, or the middle finger are most commonly affected.

**3.7** and **3.8**      Early Dupuytren's disease. The lesions are called knuckle pads (Garrod's pads).

**3.9** and **3.10**      The patient in photograph 3.9 has contractures involving only the metacarpophalangeal joints, which almost always correct after adequate surgical release. However, the proximal interphalangeal joints are also involved in the patient in photograph 3.10, and correction following surgery at these joints, and at the distal interphalangeal joints, may not be perfect. This is because the ligaments of joints with long standing contractures tend to tighten and do not always correct after fasciectomy. The soles of the feet are also affected (but the toes are not), and very occasionally there is thickening in the penile tissue (Peyronie's disease).

## Acquired

**3.11**      A ganglion, the most common swelling around the wrist.

**3.12**      A trigger thumb.

**3.13**      De Quervain's tenosynovitis. This condition involves the tendons of extensor pollicis brevis, and abductor pollicis longus. The pain of the condition is exacerbated by the manoeuvres described.

**3.14**      Spontaneous rupture of the extensor pollicis longus. Other recognised complications are carpal tunnel syndrome, Sudeck's atrophy (reflex sympathetic dystrophy), and malunion.

**3.15**      Flexor digitorum superficialis and flexor digitorum profundus to the index finger.

**3.16–3.18**      Rupture of the ulnar collateral ligament of the thumb, sometimes associated with an avulsion fracture from the base of the proximal phalanx (Photograph 3.18). This problem is commonly called

Gamekeeper's thumb because it is often found as a chronic injury said to be caused by the constant action of wringing the necks of game birds. There may be no radiological abnormalities visible, and the problem is often missed.

**3.19** Extensor pollicis longus. The deformity is often called mallet thumb, which is usually due to an avulsion fracture of the base of the distal phalanx. Occasionally it is caused by rupture of the tendon itself.

**3.20** and **3.21** He has an avulsion fracture of the volar aspect of the middle phalanx at the joint margin. The volar plate on the palmar aspect of the proximal interphalangeal joint capsule has been damaged. This prevents hyperextension, and stabilises the finger at this joint.

**3.22** A subungual haematoma has developed. A radiograph will probably show a crush fracture of the distal phalanx. In an acute case the tip of a heated paper clip through the nail evacuates the haematoma, and relieves much of the pain associated with the injury.

## Neurology

**3.23** Ulnar nerve lesion.

**3.24** The patient has true clawing of the finger: metacarpophalangeal joint hyperextension, proximal interphalangeal joint flexion, and distal interphalangeal joint flexion. These suggest a lesion of the ulnar nerve distal to its nerve supply to flexor digitorum profundus of the little finger. In the first patient the nerve lesion is more proximal as there appears to be hyperextension at the distal interphalangeal joint, which suggests that the supply to the flexor digitorum profundus is involved.

**3.25** and **3.26** The test is Froment's sign. The patient has been asked to grip the card between their thumb and the radial border of their index finger. Patients with ulnar nerve lesions may develop a paresis of the adductor pollicis and therefore cannot perform this manoeuvre without recruiting the long flexor of the thumb, which is not affected because it is usually supplied by the median nerve. A normal individual can keep their thumb straight at the interphalangeal joint when gripping a card, but the patient with an ulnar nerve lesion has to flex at the interphalangeal joint—giving a positive Froment's sign.

**3.27** and **3.28** In the left hand an abducted attitude of the little finger, and wasting of the hypothenar eminence are visible. The right hand shows marked wasting of first dorsal interosseus, and wasting patterns similar to those on the left side. The patient also shows some early clawing of the fingers of his right hand.

**3.29** Wasting of the proximal thenar eminence. Compression of the median nerve at the wrist (carpal tunnel syndrome) may be associated with paralysis of the abductor pollicis brevis (the thenar muscle almost always supplied by this nerve). This muscle often then becomes wasted.

**3.30** Psoriasis. The seronegative erosive polyarthritis which occurs in patients with psoriasis with a family history or past history of psoriasis, or with characteristic psoriatic nail changes, is called psoriatic arthritis.

**3.31**    A rheumatoid nodule.

**3.32**    Triggering of the ring and middle fingers. Rheumatoid arthritis causes any synovium within the body to become swollen and inflamed. In this woman's case the synovium that lines the flexor tendon sheath of the fingers is trapping the tendons as they glide within the tendon sheath.

**3.33**    Rheumatoid arthritis.

**3.34**    Ulnar drift.

**3.35**    Swan neck deformity.

**3.36**    The long extensors to the fingers involved have spontaneously ruptured.

**3.37** and    Heberden's nodes, which are evidence of osteoarthritis of the distal interphalangeal joints.
**3.38**

**3.39**    Gout. Tophi are present just beneath the skin. More than 90% of sufferers of chronic gout (some years' duration) show tophi in the ears, or around the joints.

**3.40**    The central slip of the extensor expansion. Untreated, this injury will result in a typical boutonnière (button hole) deformity with persistent flexion of the proximal interphalangeal joint and extension of the distal joint, as the lateral bands to the distal interphalangeal joint slide in a palmar direction.

# 4 Axial skeleton

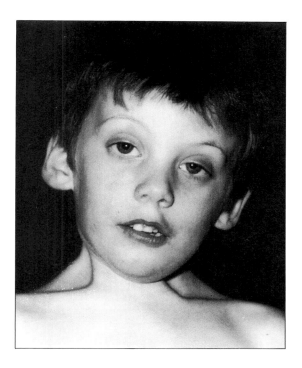

## 4.1

Describe the deformities in this boy.

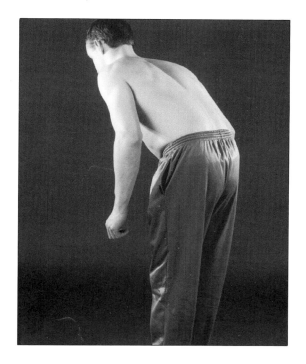

## 4.2

This patient presented with severe pain in his lower back. The total range of forward flexing motion he has is shown in the photograph. His pain is not relieved by rest.

What important spinal disorders must be excluded?

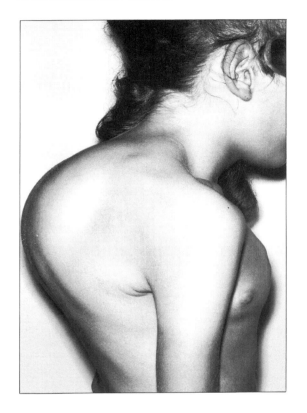

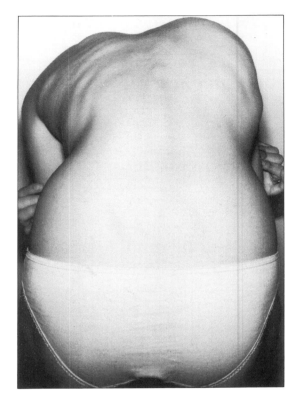

## 4.3

The young woman shown here was born with a deformed spine.

| Describe the deformity. |
| --- |

## 4.4

| What deformity does this 13 year old girl demonstrate when she bends forward? |
| --- |

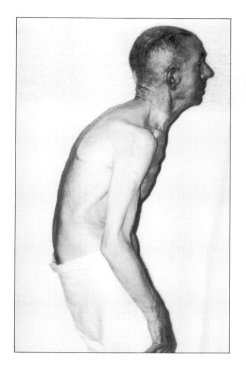

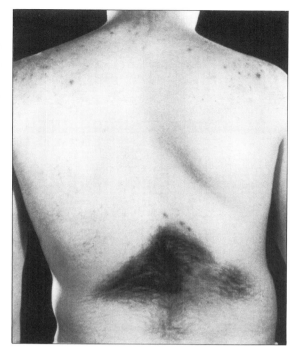

## 4.5

This elderly man has had a problem with his spine since he was 20 years old. His hip joints are also involved.

What condition does he suffer from?

## 4.6

Look at this photograph of the back of a 23 year old man.

What is the obvious physical finding?

What is the underlying disorder?

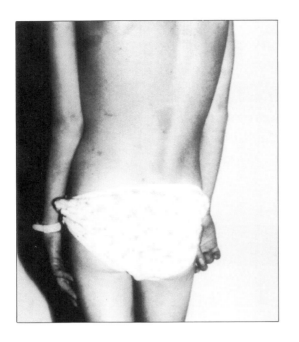 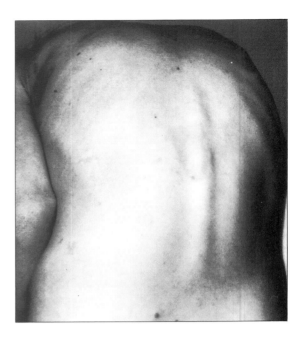

## **4.7** and **4.8**

The teenage boy in these photographs has multiple areas of pigmentation over his skin. A curvature of his spine is also apparent.

What is the underlying disorder?

What are the pigmented patches called?

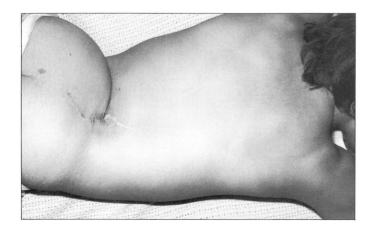

## **4.9**

What deformity is this young woman suffering from?

What is the underlying cause?

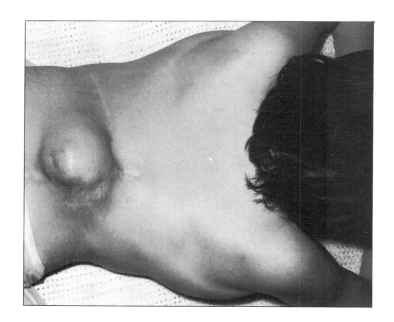

## 4.10

Describe the deformity shown here.

What is the underlying cause?

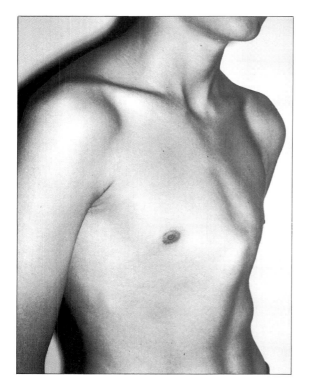

## 4.11

What is this chest deformity?

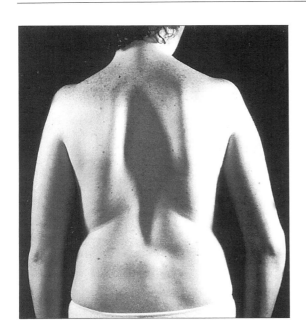

## 4.12 and 4.13

> What features are obvious on this girl's back?

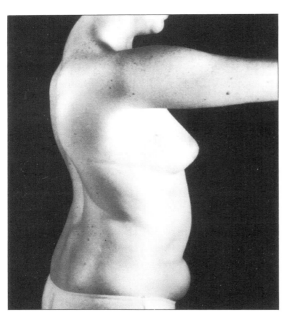

# Answers to Chapter 4

**4.1**     He has a torticollis associated with facial asymmetry.

**4.2**     Spinal infection or tumour. The patient in this case had discitis following excision of a prolapsed disc.

**4.3**     Congenital kyphosis.

**4.4**     A right rib hump associated with a thoracic scoliosis.

**4.5**     Ankylosing spondylitis, as shown by an extremely stiff spine, and a compensatory hyperlordosis of the cervical spine.

**4.6**     Physical finding: hairy patch over lumbosacral spine. Underlying disorder: spina bifida occulta, which may be associated with varying degrees of associated neurological abnormalities, for example a tethered spinal cord.

**4.7** and     Neurofibromatosis. The patches are classic café au lait spots, and are one of the cutaneous
**4.8**     manifestations of neurofibromatosis.

**4.9**     She has hyperlordosis of her spine, with a scoliosis associated with previous surgery to close a spina bifida aperta.

**4.10**     This is a kyphos secondary to spina bifida aperta.

**4.11**     Pectus carinatum. A pigeon deformity of the chest results from undue prominence of the sternum with lateral flattening of the chest wall. The opposite deformity is pectus excavatum, or funnel chest. Asymmetric pectus carinatum may be a marker for underlying disease.

**4.12** and     There is a step at the lumbosacral junction, and the sacrum appears long. This is typical of
**4.13**     spondylolisthesis, a slipping forward of one vertebra on another at the level of L5 over the body of the sacrum.

# 5 Hip and pelvis

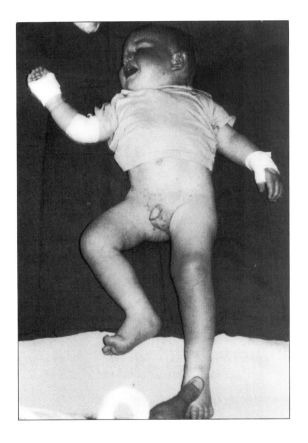

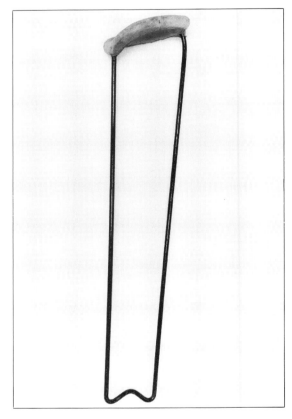

## 5.1

This 5 month old baby was generally unwell. On admission to hospital he had a high temperature, was toxic, and any attempt to move his right leg caused him extreme discomfort.

What is your differential diagnosis?

## 5.2

What is the name of this splint?

What is it commonly used for?

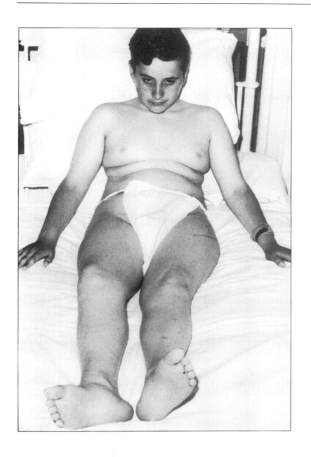

## 5.3

This 14 year old boy suffered discomfort in his right knee, and had a limp for 2–3 months before referral to hospital.

What is the probable diagnosis?

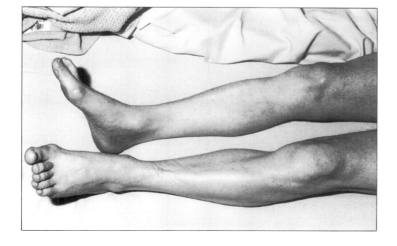

## 5.4

A 65 year old man fell in the street and was admitted to hospital with the physical sign shown in the photograph.

What is the physical sign?

What is the probable diagnosis?

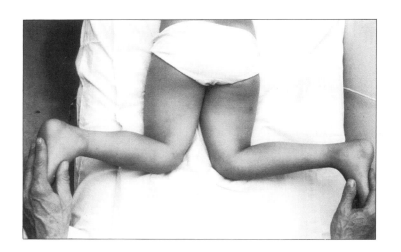

## 5.5

This young girl walks with bilateral intoeing gait.

---
**What is the cause of this?**
---

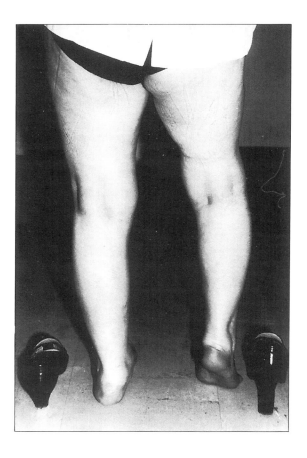

## 5.6

The femur of this woman had been fractured previously.

---
**What has been the outcome of this fracture?**
---

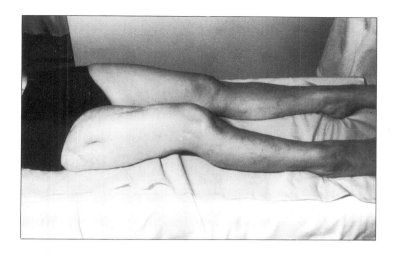

## 5.7 and 5.8

> What physical sign does this patient demonstrate?

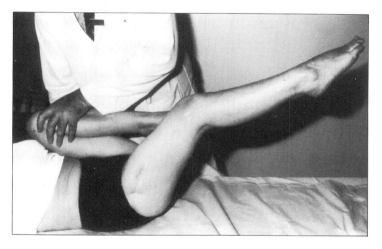

> What is the test called?

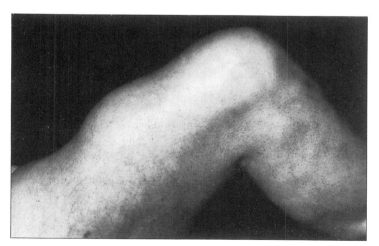

## 5.9

This middle aged man presented with a swelling over the anterior aspect of his right thigh. The swelling was painless, hard, and fixed to muscle (not bone).

> What diagnosis is likely?

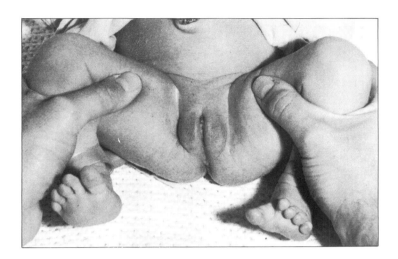

## 5.10

What test is being performed on this baby?

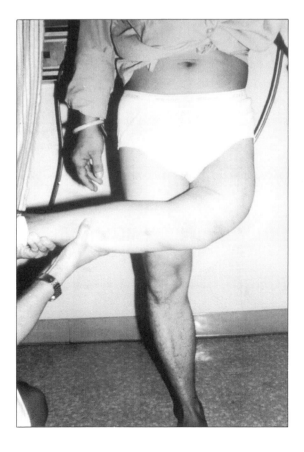

## 5.11

What is wrong with this patient's thigh?

# Answers to Chapter 5

**5.1**    Septic arthritis; in this case septic arthritis of the right hip.

**5.2**    A Thomas splint, which was introduced by Hugh Owen Thomas (1834–1891) of Liverpool. The Thomas splint is commonly used in treating femoral fractures or inflammation of the knee.

**5.3**    Slipped right femoral capital epiphysis; note the physical appearance of the patient.

**5.4**    Shortening and external rotation of the right leg secondary to a fracture of the right femoral neck.

**5.5**    Excessive femoral anteversion, or persistent fetal anteversion. This is demonstrated by excessive range of internal rotation when the patient lies prone.

**5.6**    The patient's leg has shortened, probably secondary to a malunion. As a consequence, she walks on the ball of her foot and needs a significant shoe raise.

**5.7** and    Fixed flexion deformity of the right hip. The test is Thomas's hip flexion.
**5.8**

**5.9**    Soft tissue sarcoma.

**5.10**    Ortolani's test, used to screen neonates for congenital hip dislocation. The test is positive if a dislocated hip reduces with a marked 'clunk' (not a 'click').

**5.11**    He has a long established pseudoarthritis in his left femoral shaft. (Picture by kind permission of Professor P. Balasubramamian, Singapore).

# 6  Knee

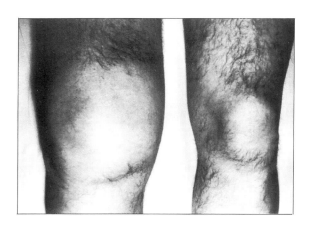

## 6.1

This 22 year old footballer had sustained an injury to his right knee while on the field. He had had no previous problems with his right knee and the photograph was taken within half an hour of the injury.

> What is the clinical diagnosis?
>
> What are the probable underlying causes?

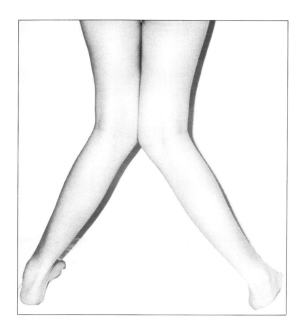

## 6.2

> Describe this deformity.

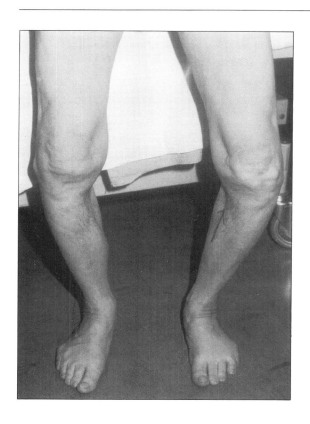

## 6.3

The knees of this man are painful. The pain is worse in the left knee than in the right.

Describe the deformity.

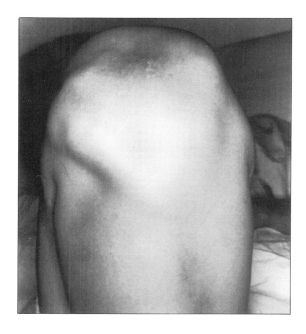

## 6.4

What is wrong with this knee?

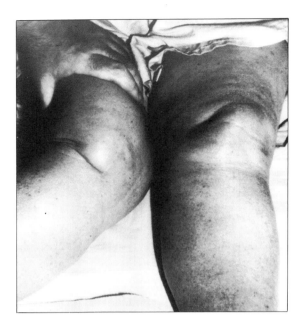

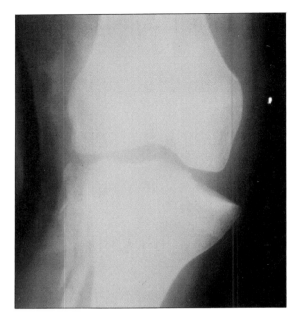

## **6.5** and **6.6**

A woman fell and injured her right knee. Under anaesthesia the manoeuvre shown in Photograph 6.5 could be performed by valgus strain of the knee.

**What structures do you think she has damaged?**

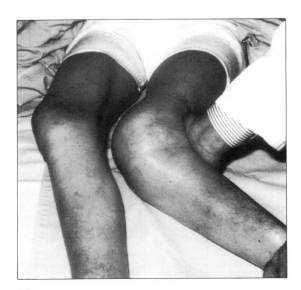

## **6.7**

This woman has instability of the knee associated with a long standing joint problem.

**What is the underlying disease?**

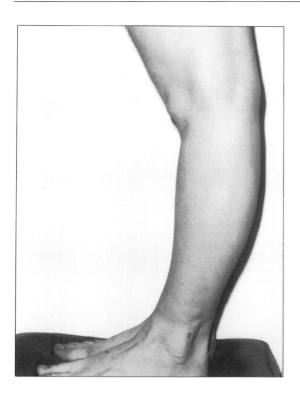

## 6.8

Describe the deformity in this 18 year old patient.

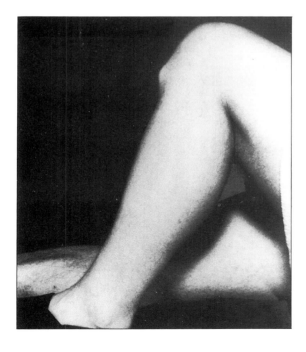

## 6.9

What condition did this young man have as an adolescent?

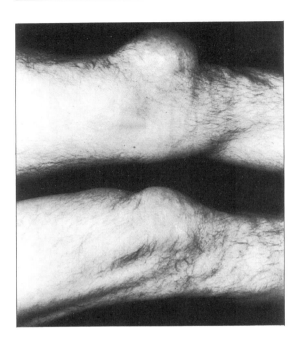

## 6.10

The patient in this photograph has developed a swelling in his left knee.

> **What is it called?**
>
> **What could the cause be?**

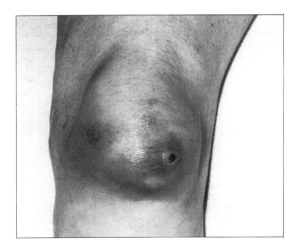

## 6.11

This patient has a condition similar to that shown in the previous photograph.

> **What has happened?**

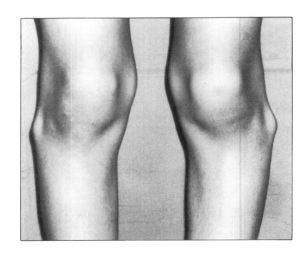

## 6.12

Prominent swellings are visible on the posterior lateral aspects of the knees of this patient.

> **What is the cause of these swellings?**

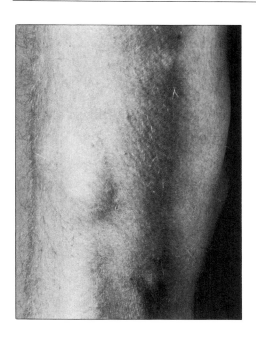

## 6.13

A swelling at the posterior aspect of the right knee. The knee is stiff and occasionally painful.

> **What is the swelling?**

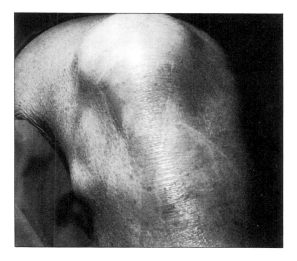

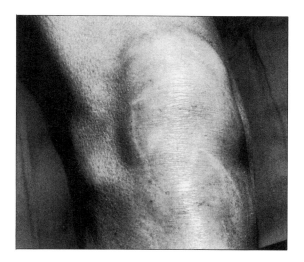

## 6.14 and 6.15

This man has had pain over the lateral aspect of his right knee. A swelling, which transilluminated, became apparent on the outer border of the knee, just below the joint line. On extension of the knee the cyst became less apparent.

> **What is the probable diagnosis?**

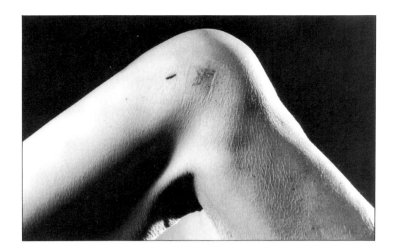

## 6.16 and 6.17

The right knee of this rugby player was injured in a head on tackle. The first photograph shows the position of his knee when flexed at 90°; Photograph 6.17 demonstrates a further physical sign.

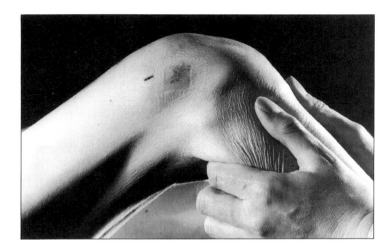

> What are these physical signs?

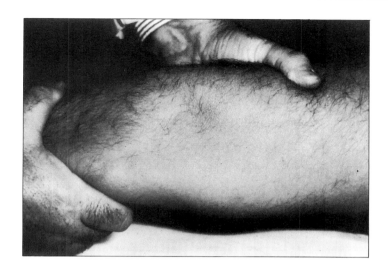

## 6.18 and 6.19

What test is being performed here?

Which structure is being tested?

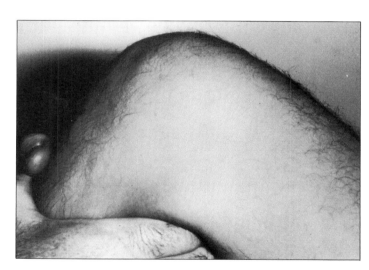

# Answers to Chapter 6

**6.1**     Hemiarthrosis of the right knee. There is obvious swelling of the suprapatellar pouch, and the hollows normally present on the medial and lateral aspects of the patellar ligament are bulging. The probable causes are rupture of the anterior or posterior cruciate ligaments, peripheral detachment of either meniscus, or an intra-articular fracture.

**6.2**     Knock knee, or genu valgum. The cause in the UK is more likely to be renal rather than nutritional rickets. Idiopathic knock knee does not become as gross as that in this photograph.

**6.3**     Genu varum, in this case secondary to osteoarthritis which is largely affecting the medial compartment of the knee. Genu varum is often a late sequel of medial meniscectomy.

**6.4**     The patella has dislocated laterally when the knee flexed. (Picture by kind permission of Professor P. Balsasubramamian.)

**6.5** and     The patient has ruptured the medial collateral ligament of her knee and, because the knee opens on
**6.6**     valgus straining in extension, this is associated with rupture of one or both cruciate ligaments. The stress radiograph (Photograph 6.6) shows marked opening of the knee on valgus strain with an associated fracture of the upper fibula.

**6.7**     Rheumatoid arthritis.

**6.8**     Hyperextension of the knee, or genu recurvatum. This may be a result of generalised joint laxity, or may follow an epiphyseal injury.

**6.9**     Osgood Schlatter's disease. Note the permanent bony prominence of the tibial tuberosity.

**6.10**     Prepatellar bursitis (housemaid's knee). This condition is usually associated with occupations such as carpet fitting.

**6.11**     The prepatellar bursa has become infected and has discharged.

**6.12**     Congenital dislocation of the proximal tibiofibular joint.

**6.13**     A popliteal cyst associated with an arthritic process in the knee. The cyst may be shown on arthrography.

**6.14** and     Lateral meniscal cyst. This does not always require treatment, depending on the severity of the
**6.15**     symptoms.

**6.16** and     Photograph 6.16 shows 'back knee', which is commonly seen in ruptures of the posterior cruciate
**6.17**     ligament. Photograph 6.17 demonstrates relocation of the tibia on the femur by a draw test. Following posterior cruciate ruptures the tibial plateau tends to glide posteriorly on the femoral condyles with the knee flexed at 90°, and can be relocated as demonstrated in this photograph.

**6.18** and     Lachman's test. This test is commonly performed to assess the competence of the anterior cruciate
**6.19**     ligament. If positive it may be verified by an anterior draw test, as shown in Photograph 6.19. The examiner usually sits on the patient's foot to stabilise the leg.

# 7 Lower leg/tibia

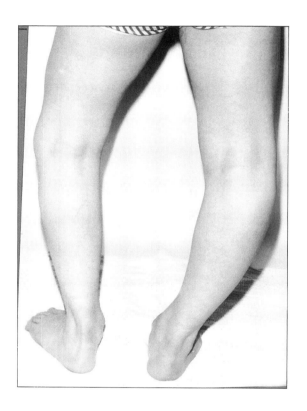

## 7.1

> Describe this deformity.

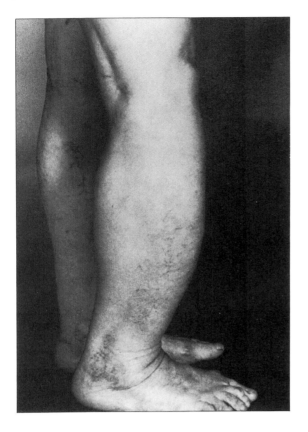 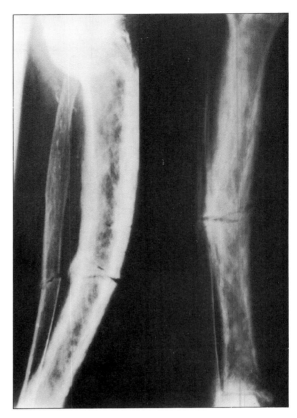

## 7.2 and 7.3

This elderly man has a deformity of his right shin which causes him pain. His thigh is also deformed, and he is deaf.

What condition does he suffer from?

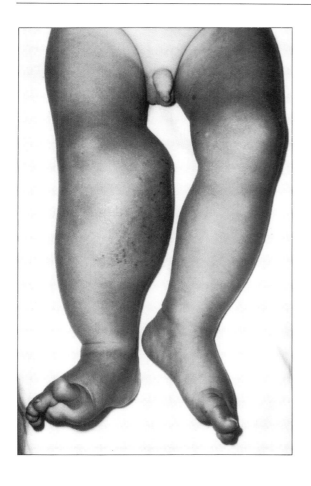

## 7.4

The right leg of this baby became swollen soon after birth. The swelling has increased in size and has caused a significant discrepancy in leg lengths.

| What could the swelling be? |
| --- |

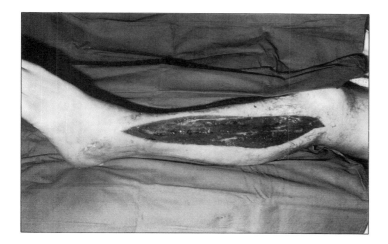

## 7.5

The patient shown here fractured his tibia and developed severe pain in his left leg. He had to be treated surgically as an emergency.

| What operation has been performed? |
| --- |

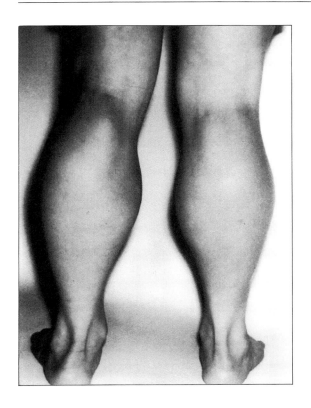

## 7.6

This boy had an older brother who suffered from the same condition and died in his teens.

> **What condition do they both suffer from?**
>
> **What does this photograph demonstrate?**

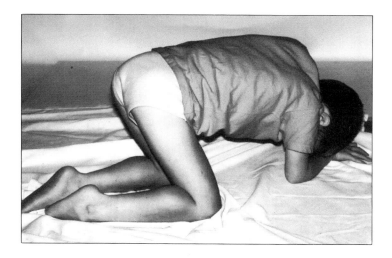

## 7.7

> **What is this boy trying to do?**

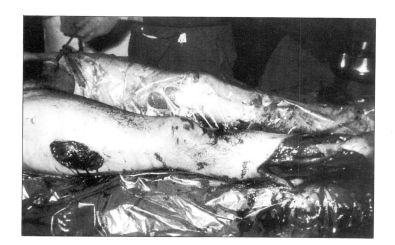

## 7.8

Describe the injuries to the leg shown here.

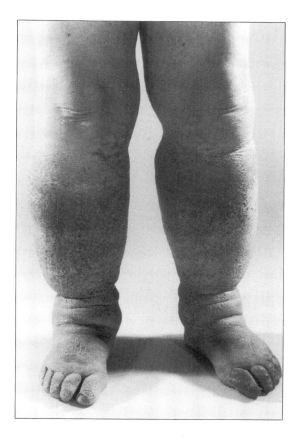

## 7.9

Describe this condition.

# Answers to Chapter 7

**7.1**    Tibia vara (Blount's disease)—progressive varus deformity of the upper end of the tibia. This deformity is most common in infancy, but occasionally occurs in adolescence. It may be unilateral or bilateral, and usually occurs in Negroes.

**7.2** and **7.3**    Paget's disease. The deformity of the tibia may become increasingly painful because of the condition itself, and also because stress fractures occur in the bone as the deformity increases, as seen on the radiograph.

**7.4**    The development of a leg length discrepancy suggests that the lesion is hypervascular. The lesion in this case is a congenital arteriovenous malformation, which causes excessive stimulation of the growth plate around the knee and causes accelerated axial growth. Note the obvious small vessels in the skin on the inner side of the baby's calf.

**7.5**    The patient has undergone a fasciotomy and debridement of the anterior compartment of his leg, because a compartment syndrome has occurred secondary to his tibial fracture. Pain in a fracture patient immobilised in a plaster cast needs careful evaluation to exclude a compartment syndrome. Other important symptoms are paraesthesia and difficulty in moving the digits.

**7.6**    The pseudohypertrophy of the calf muscles suggests Duchenne muscular dystrophy.

**7.7**    He is attempting to stand starting from a supine position on the floor. This is Gower's Test, which is used to assess the strength of the muscles of a patient with Duchenne muscular dystrophy.

**7.8**    Compound fracture of the tibia and femur.

**7.9**    Chronic lymphoedema of the lower limbs. Various degrees of lymphoedema can occur, ranging from the mildest slight swelling around an ankle to this gross swelling. Lymphatic insufficiency may become obvious only after an injury and marked local damage.

# **8** Foot

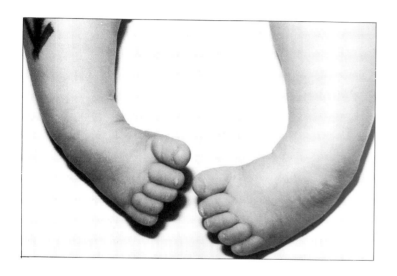

## **8.1** and **8.2**

This child was born with deformed feet.

> What is the condition called?
>
> What are the three main components of the deformity?

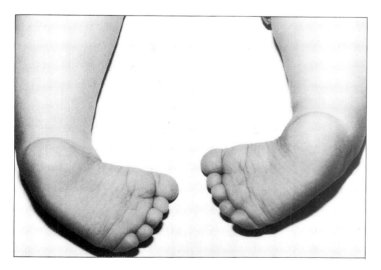

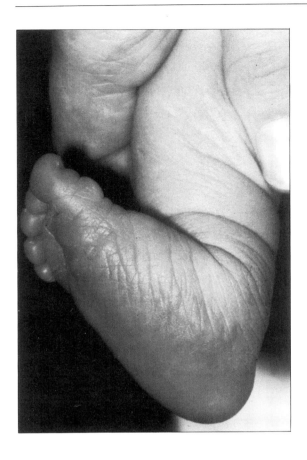

## 8.3 and 8.4

At delivery a baby was found to have the foot deformity shown in Photograph 3.

---

What is the name of the deformity?

What other condition is associated with it in 5–10% of infants?

---

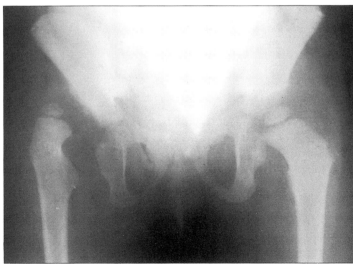

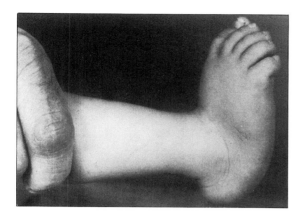

## **8.5** and **8.6**

This foot deformity persisted in a 6 month old infant.

> What is the deformity?
>
> Name two conditions that can be associated with it.

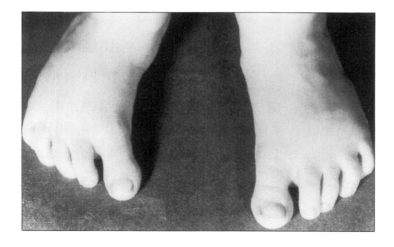

## **8.7**

The foot deformity shown was noted when this child started walking. The ankle and hindfoot are normal.

> What is the deformity?
>
> What is the natural history of the condition?

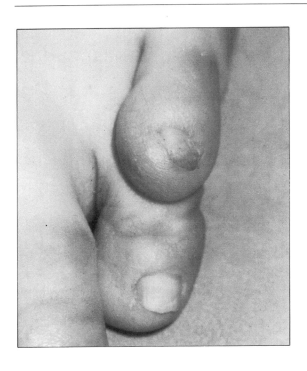

## 8.8

This deformity is commonly seen in orthopaedic practice.

> **What is it called?**

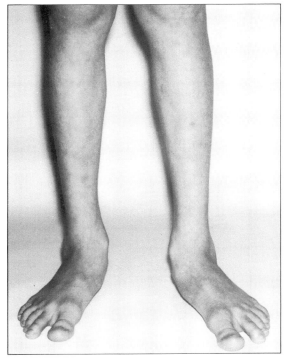

## 8.9, 8.10 and 8.11

This 13 year old boy has had feet of this shape since infancy.

> **What is the correct name for this condition?**

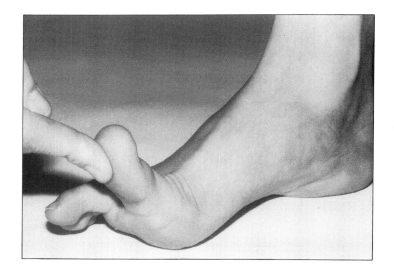

What test is being performed here?

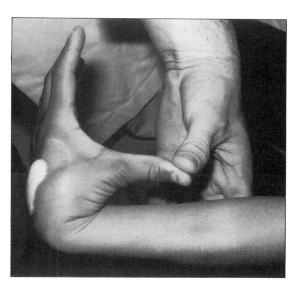

What does this test signify?

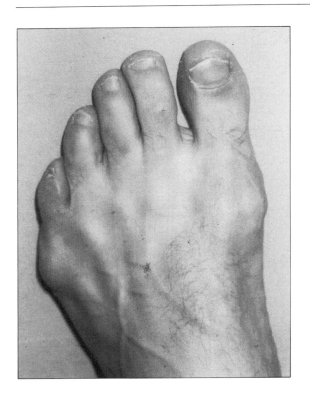

## 8.12

This patient complained that the lateral border of his foot was rubbing in his shoe.

> **What deformity is present?**

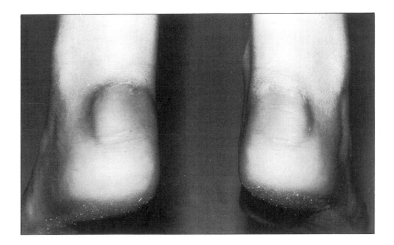

## 8.13

This teenage girl complained of pain in the back of her heels when she wore certain types of shoes.

> **What is the cause of her pain?**

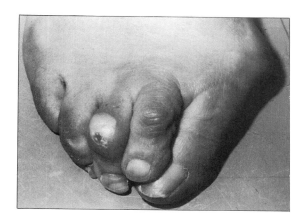

## 8.14

Several toe deformities are shown here.

> Name two of them.

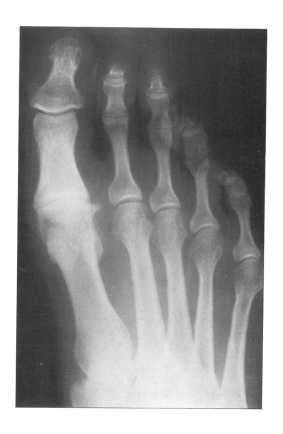

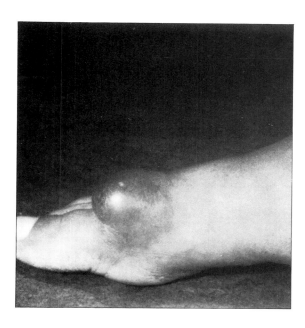

## 8.15 and 8.16

This patient complained of pain in the great toe when walking.

> What disorder does he show?
>
> What is the cystic lesion on the dorsum of the foot?

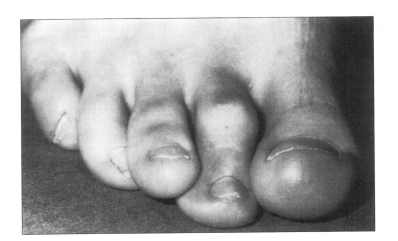

## 8.17

This elderly patient has a painful second toe.

> **What is the deformity?**

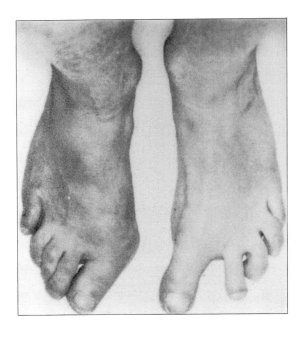

## 8.18

Following surgery for a bunion this woman developed a deformity of the left great toe.

> **What is it called?**

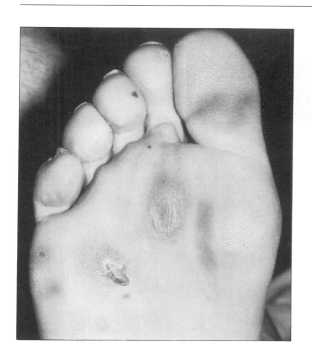

## 8.19

Two specific areas on the sole of his foot were causing this patient pain.

> What is the lesion under the second metatarsal head?
>
> What is the lesion under the fourth metatarsal head?

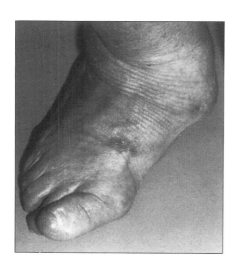

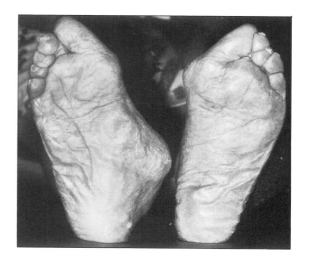

## 8.20 and 8.21

This woman has a generalised joint condition (arthropathy). When walking she experiences severe pain in the balls of her feet.

> What is the underlying disorder?
>
> Why does she feel pain in her forefeet?

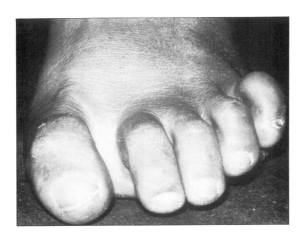

## 8.22

> What deformity of the toes is shown here?

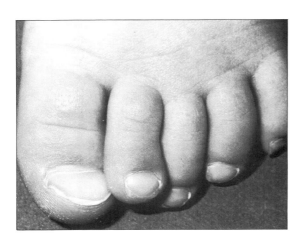

## 8.23

> What is this minor deformity of the second toe known as?

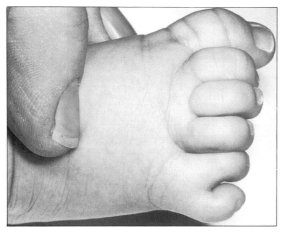

## 8.24

This baby was born with the toe deformity shown here.

> What is the correct term for the condition?

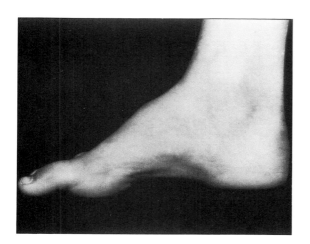

## **8.25** and **8.26**

Both feet of this young man are painful.

---
**What condition does he have?**
---

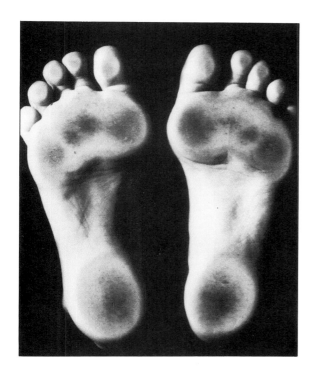

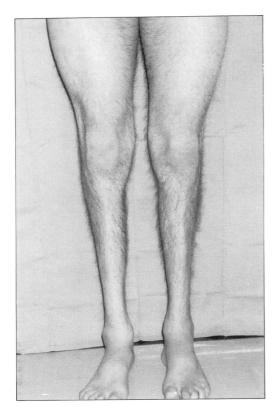

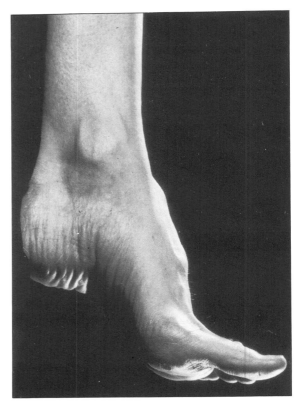

## 8.27

The teenager shown here has the same foot condition as the previous patient (8.26). His father and uncle also suffered with the problem. He has already undergone surgery to his feet.

> **What could the underlying condition be?**

## 8.28

This adolescent girl has the foot condition described in the previous two cases. She is very tall for her age and is slim. She also has scoliosis and hypermobile joints.

> **What condition does she suffer from?**

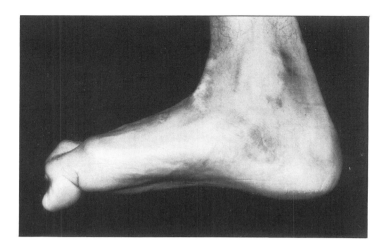

## 8.29 and 8.30

Two years ago this patient suffered a tibial fracture, which was followed by severe calf pain. His foot later became stiff.

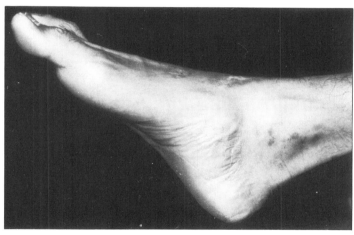

> What is the foot deformity called?
>
> What underlying problem in his lower leg has caused this foot deformity?

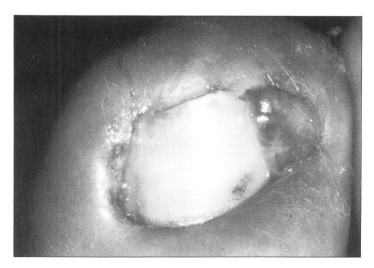

## 8.31

> What is the problem on the medial nail fold?

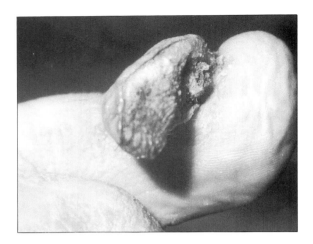

## 8.32

| What toenail deformity is seen here? |

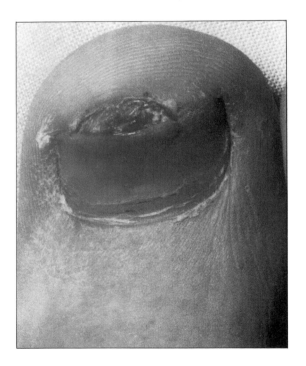

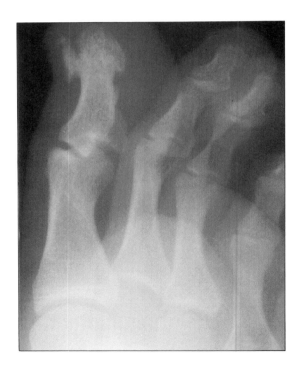

## 8.33 and 8.34

This patient complained about a painful lesion under the nail of his great toe.

| What causes the pain? |

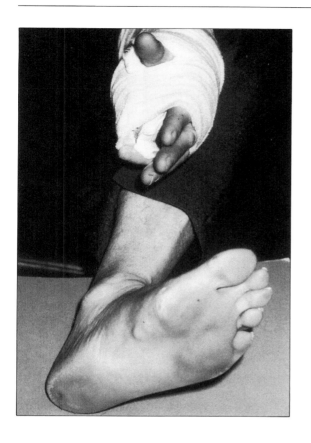

## 8.35

This patient noticed a swelling on the medial aspect of the sole of the foot. He has recently had a similar lesion excised from his left little finger.

---

**What is the condition called?**

---

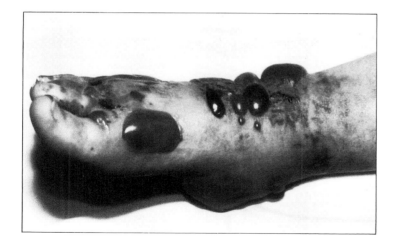

## 8.36

This foot was run over by a car. The foot looked like this 24 hours after the injury.

---

**What are these lesions called?**

**How might you prevent them from developing when the patient initially attends the hospital?**

---

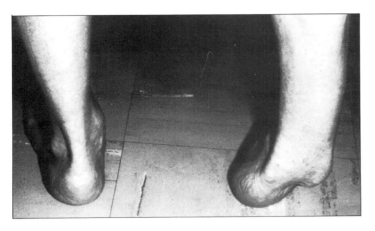

## 8.37 and 8.38

This man had injured his right ankle as a child.

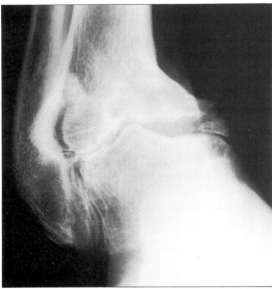

> **How would you describe the deformity?**
>
> **What is the common name given to this injury?**

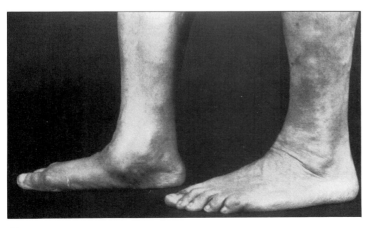

## 8.39 and 8.40

This middle aged woman developed pain and swelling on the inner aspect of her right ankle behind the medial malleolus. Over the following weeks she noticed increasing deformity of the foot.

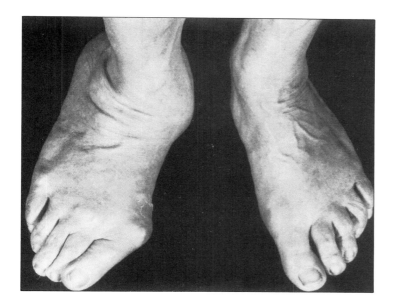

How would you describe the foot?

What is the probable diagnosis in a woman of this age?

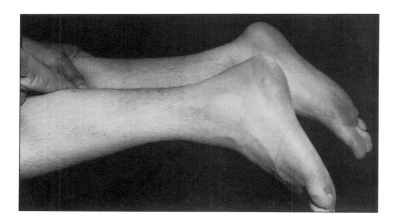

## 8.41

This test is performed by squeezing the patients' calf while they lie prone.

What is the test called?

If the result is positive what should happen?

What does a positive result signify?

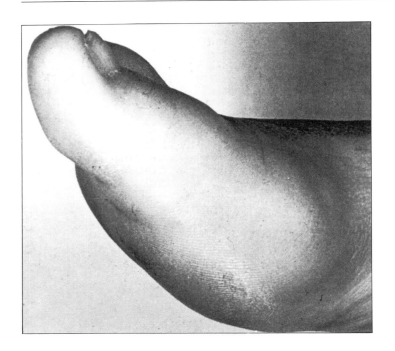

## 8.42

This great toe was acutely swollen and painful at the metatarsophalangeal joint. The overlying skin was shiny and red.

> **What is the most common cause of this painful condition?**

# Answers to Chapter 8

**8.1** and **8.2** Congenital talipes equinovarus (clubfoot), one of the most common congenital deformities. The three main components are equinus of the ankle, varus of the heel, and adduction of the forefoot. The condition is more common in boys than girls, occurring in 1–2 live births in 1000.

**8.3** and **8.4** The child has a calcaneo valgus deformity. Congenital dislocation of the hip (now often called developmental dysplasia of the hip) may be associated with this deformity, as demonstrated in Photograph 8.4.

**8.5** and **8.6** Congenital vertical talus. Conditions that may be associated with this problem are arthrogryposis and spinal dysraphism.

**8.7** Metatarsus varus or metatarsus adducts which, in the vast majority of children, corrects spontaneously. It tends to be a self limiting condition and most children suffering from it have normal feet by the age of 5 years: only about 10% need surgical correction because their feet are rigid and do not passively correct to neutral.

**8.8** Overriding fifth toe or varus little toe, which is often asymptomatic.

**8.9–8.11** The condition is mobile pes planus (also called mobile flatfoot deformity). The test being performed is Jack's test (or the great toe extension test). On passive dorsiflexion of the great toe at the first metatarsaophalangeal joint the patient's arch develops, and helps to distinguish this condition from a rigid flatfoot deformity. A positive test result indicates that, although when standing there is no arch, the arch mechanism is functioning normally. The low thumb/forearm index shown in Photograph 8.11 indicates that these patients have hypermobile or lax joints.

**8.12** A bunionette, a bony prominence on the lateral aspect of the fifth metatarsal head. It is covered by a bursa, in the same way as a hallux valgus.

**8.13** Heel bumps, also called 'pump bumps', or 'winter heel', caused by prominence of the superior angle of the calcaneum. They are occasionally associated with a bursa over the bony prominence. The condition is usually seen in young adults.

**8.14** Deformities include hallux valgus, hammer toe, and overriding toes.

**8.15** and **8.16** The disorder is hallux rigidus. The patient has a dorsal bunion, which is diagnostic of this condition.

**8.17** Hammer toe—flexion of the proximal interphalangeal joint, extension of the distal interphalangeal joint, and a neutral or extended metatarsophalangeal joint. The second toe is the digit most commonly involved.

**8.18** Hallux varus. This deformity causes more discomfort when wearing shoes than hallux valgus.

**8.19** The lesion under the second metatarsal head is a callosity caused by pressure from an underlying bony prominence. A verruca, or plantar wart, caused by a viral infection is visible under the fourth metatarsal head.

**8.20** and **8.21**    Rheumatoid arthritis. The inflamed synovium has destroyed the metatarsophalangeal joints and the plantar plates. Because of this subluxation of the joint and dorsal displacement of the toes are occurring, and the metatarsal heads are exposed to excess pressure on the sole of the foot.

**8.22**    Claw toe, which in this patient followed poliomyelitis. The toe is flexed at both the proximal and the distal interphalangeal joints. The metatarsophalangeal joint may be neutral or extended.

**8.23**    Curly toes, which occur in young children. The condition is best left untreated until the foot has stopped growing. If symptoms persist at that stage treatment may be necessary.

**8.24**    Polydactyly (multiple digits).

**8.25** and **8.26**    Pes cavus.

**8.27**    Charcot–Marie–Tooth disease, or peroneal muscular atrophy. (Hereditary motor and sensory neuropathy Type 1.)

**8.28**    Marfan's syndrome.

**8.29** and **8.30**    The deformity is Volkmann's ischaemic contracture. An acute, unrecognised (and therefore untreated) compartment syndrome of the lower leg musculature has caused fibrosis of the muscles and shortening of the muscle tendons, and thus the toe deformities. The deformities are fixed in the plantigrade position but disappear on plantarflexion of the ankle.

**8.31**    Ingrowing toenail.

**8.32**    Onychogryphosis.

**8.33** and **8.34**    Subungual exostosis.

**8.35**    Dupuytren's contracture. The lesion in the foot always recurs, so surgery is not helpful here.

**8.36**    Fracture blisters. Elevation of the injured limb in a splint will help keep the swelling to a minimum and prevent these lesions forming.

**8.37** and **8.38**    Varus deformity of the ankle/distal tibia, often called a railing fracture because of the mechanism of production of the injury. It is caused by an injury to the distal growth plate of the tibia in childhood.

**8.39** and **8.40**    The arch has flattened spontaneously and the instep collapsed. It is probably caused by rupture of the tibialis posterior tendon, which sometimes occurs spontaneously in middle aged patients.

**8.41**    The test is Simmond's or Thompson's test. A passive plantar flex of the ankle should occur on squeezing the calf. Failure of the ankle to passively plantar flex suggests that there has been a rupture of the Achilles tendon.

**8.42**    Acute gout. Urate crystals will be found in the synovial fluid of the joint, and the level of uric acid in the serum may be raised.

# **9** Miscellaneous conditions

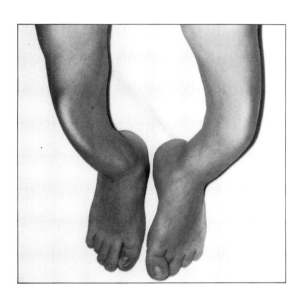

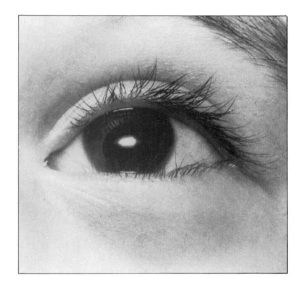

## **9.1** and **9.2**

The limbs of this 6 year old boy are markedly deformed. Also, the whites of his eyes are discoloured.

What condition does he suffer from?

What is the anomaly that can be seen in his eye?

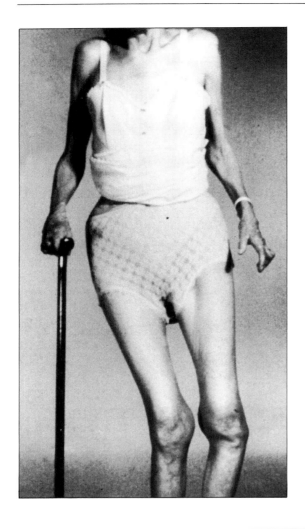

## 9.3

What condition does this woman suffer from?

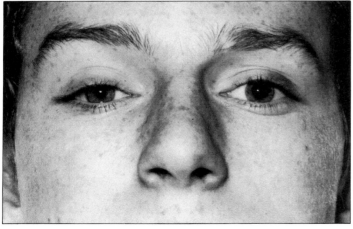

## 9.4

This patient was injured in a motor-cycle accident. He developed wasting of his right arm and a right sided facial deformity.

What injury has he sustained?

What is the associated facial problem called?

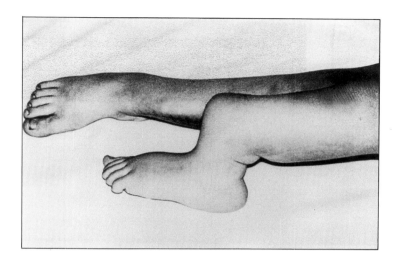

# 9.5 and 9.6

This child was born with a progressive deformity of the left shin. The child went on to develop a spinal deformity. The marked anterior bowing in the leg is typical of a severe deformity.

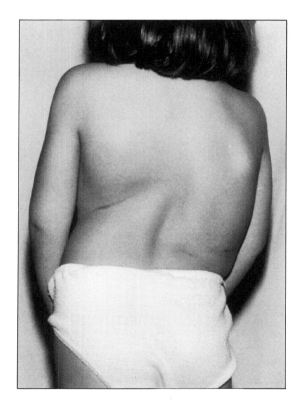

What is the underlying disorder?

What is the deformity of the tibia?

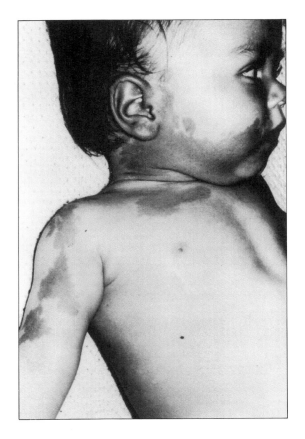 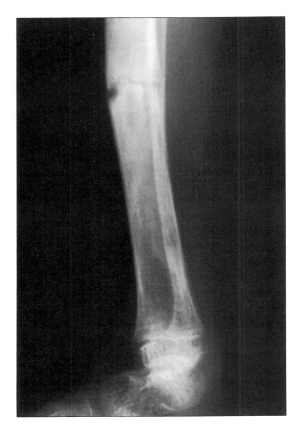

## **9.7** and **9.8**

This child was born with abnormal skin pigmentation. Bone deformities subsequently developed, and his bones tended to spontaneously fracture.

What condition does this child suffer from?

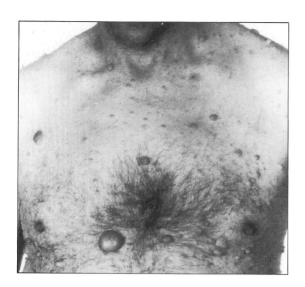

## 9.9

> What are the lesions on this man's skin?

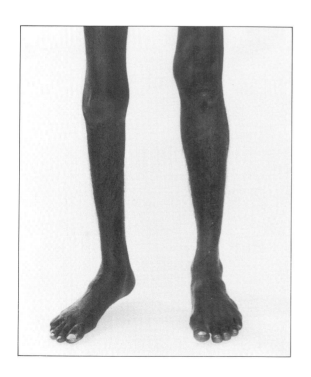

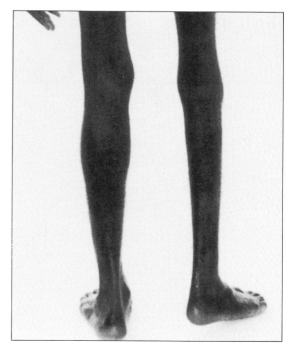

## 9.10 and 9.11

This woman suffered a viral infection as a child which has left her with a shortened, wasted right leg.

> What condition has she suffered from?

# Answers to Chapter 9

**9.1** and  Osteogenesis imperfecta, associated with blue sclera.
**9.2**

**9.3**  Rheumatoid arthritis. Note the deformities in her hands, and the 'windswept knees' with right genu valgum and left genu varum.

**9.4**  The patient has injured his brachial plexus. The injury is associated with a right sided Horner's syndrome (miosis, enophthalmos and anhidrosis). (Photograph by kind permission of Mr R. Birch.)

**9.5** and  Neurofibromatosis and pseudoarthrosis of the tibia. Scoliosis may also be a feature of the disease.
**9.6**

**9.7** and  Albright's syndrome. This condition is associated with polyosteotic fibrous dysplasia and skin
**9.8**  pigmentation. Precocious puberty occurs in girls.

**9.9**  Neurofibromas. The patient suffers from neurofibromatosis, which is characterised by café-au-lait patches, tumours of nerve trunks, overgrowth of tissues, and various skeletal deformities.

**9.10** and  Poliomyelitis. Fortunately this condition is now relatively rare because of the success of immunisation.
**9.11**  Poliomyelitis is purely a motor nerve lesion, causing no sensory changes.

# Index

*Page numbers in brackets refer to answers*

Achilles tendon rupture   8.41, (84)
Acromioclavicular joint dislocation   1.8, 1.9, (11)
Albright's syndrome   9.7, 9.8, (90)
Ankle deformity   8.37, 8.38, 8.39, (84)
Ankylosing spondylitis   4.5, (43)
Arteriovenous malformation   7.4, (64)
Arthritis *See also* rheumatoid arthritis
   osteoarthritis   3.37, 3.38, (36)
   psoriatic   3.30, (35)
   septic   1.15, (11), 5.1, (49)
Axillary nerve palsy   1.16, (11)

"Back" knee   6.16, 6.17, (58)
Back pain   4.2, (43)
Biceps rupture   1.7, (11)
Blount's disease   7.1, (64)
Boutonnière deformity   3.40, (36)
Brachial plexus injury   9.4, (90)
Bunion, dorsal   8.15, (83)
Bunionette   8.12, (83)
Bursa
   infected,   6.11, (58)
   subdeltoid   1.22, (11)
Bursitis
   prepatellar   6.10, (58)
   subacromial   1.19, (11)

Cafe au lait spots   4.7, 4.8, (43)
Calcaneo valgus deformity   8.3, (83)
Calf muscle pseudohypertrophy   7.6, (64)
Callosity   8.19, (83)
Campodactyly   3.5, 3.6, (34)
Carpal tunnel syndrome   3.29, (35)
Charcot-Marie-Tooth disease   8.27, (84)
Chest deformity   4.11, (43)
Clavicular fracture   1.6, (11)
Claw fingers   3.24, 3.27, 3.28, (35)

Claw toe   8.22, (84)
Clubfoot   8.1, 8.2, (83)
Compartment syndrome   7.5, (64), 8.29, 8.30, (84)
Compound fracture   7.8, (64)
Congenital dislocation of hip   5.10, (49), 8.4, (83)
Cubitus valgus   2.9, (16)
Cubitus varus   2.1, (16)
Curly toes   8.23, (84)
Cyst
   meniscal   6.14, 6.15, (58)
   popliteal   6.13, (58)

Deltoid muscle wasting   1.17, 1.18, 1.21, (11)
De Quervain's tenosynovitis   3.13, (34)
Diaphysial aclasis   2.7, (16)
Discitis   4.2, (43)
Drop wrist   2.3, (16)
Duchenne muscular dystrophy   7.6, 7.7, (64)
Dupuytren's disease   3.7, 3.8, 3.9, 3.10, (34), 8.35, (84)

Elbow
   hyperextension   2.6, (16)
   posterior dislocation   2.10, (16)
Exostoses, hereditary multiple   2.7, (16)
Exostosis, subungual   8.33, 8.34, (84)
Extensor pollicis longus
   damage   3.19, (35)
   spontaneous rupture   3.14, (34)
Eye anomaly   9.2, (90)

Facioscapulo humeral dystrophy   1.13, 1.14, (11)
Fasciotomy   7.5, (64)
Fingers
   boutonnière deformity   3.40, (36)
   clawing   3.24, 3.27, 3.28, (35)
   damage to flexors   3.15, (34)
   rupture of long extensors   3.36, (36)

subungual haematoma   3.22, (35)
swan neck deformity   3.35, (36)
triggering   3.32, (36)
Femoral neck fracture   5.4, (49)
Femur
    anteversion   5.5, (49)
    fracture   5.6, (49), 7.8, (64)
    pseudoarthritis   5.11, (49)
    slipped capital epiphysis   5.3, (49)
Flatfoot deformity, mobile   8.9, 8.10, (83)
Fracture blisters   8.36, (84)
Froment's sign   3.25, 3.26, (35)

Gamekeeper's thumb   3.16, 3.17, 3.18, (34–35)
Ganglion   3.11, (34)
Garrod's pads   3.8, (34)
Genu recurvatum   6.8, (58)
Genu valgum   6.2, (58)
Genu varum   6.3, (58)
Gout   3.39, (36), 8.42, (84)
Gower's Test   7.7, (64)
Granuloma, infected   3.2, (34)

Hallux rigidus   8.15, 8.16, (83)
Hallux valgus   8.14, (83)
Hallux varus   8.18, (83)
Hammer toe   8.14, 8.17, (83)
Heberden's nodes   3.37, 3.38, (36)
Heel bumps   8.13, (83)
Hip
    congenital dislocation   5.10, (49), 8.4, (83)
    fixed flexion deformity   5.7, 5.8, (49)
    fracture   5.4, (49)
Horner's syndrome   9.4, (90)
Housemaid's knee   6.10, (58)
Humerus
    congenital amputation   1.11, (11)
    radiography   1.3, (11)
Hyperlordosis   4.9, (43)

Ingrowing toenail   8.31, (84)

Jack's test   8.10, (83)
Joint hypermobility   2.6, (16), 8.11, (83)

Knee
    "back knee"   6.16, 6.17, (58)

hemiarthrosis   6.1, (58)
hyperextension   6.8, (58)
rheumatoid arthritis   6.7, (58), 9.3, (90)
Knee ligaments
    anterior cruciate: competence   6.18, 6.19, (58)
    medial collateral: rupture   6.5, 6.6, (58)
    posterior cruciate: rupture   6.16, 6.17, (58)
Knock knee   6.2, (58)
Knuckle pads   3.8, (34)
Kyphos   4.10, (43)
Kyphosis   4.3, (43)

Lachman's test   6.18, (58)
Leg length discrepancy   5.6, (49), 9.10, 9.11, (90)
    infants   7.4, (64)
Lipoma   1.20, (11)
Lobster hands   3.3, (34)
Lymphoedema   7.9, (64)

Mallet thumb   3.19, (35)
Marfan's syndrome   8.28, (84)
Meniscus, lateral: cyst   6.14, 6.15, (58)
Metatarsus varus   8.7, (83)
Mobile pes planus   8.9, 8.10, (83)

Neuralgic amyotrophy   1.12, (11)
Neurofibromatosis   4.7, 4.8, (43), 9.5, 9.6, 9.9, (90)

Onychogryphosis   8.32, (84)
Ortolani's test   5.10, (49)
Osteoarthritis   3.37, 3.38, (36)
Osgood Schlatter's disease   6.9, (58)
Osteogenesis imperfecta   9.1, 9.2, (90)

Paget's disease   7.2, 7.3, (64)
Patellar dislocation   6.4, (58)
Pectus carinatum   4.11, (43)
Peroneal muscular atrophy   8.27, (84)
Pes cavus   8.25, 8.26, (84)
Phalangeal fractures   3.20, 3.21, 3.22, (35)
Phocomelia   1.11, (11)
Pigeon chest   4.11, (43)
Plantar wart   8.19, (83)
Poliomyelitis   9.10, 9.11, (90)
Polydactyly   8.24, (84)
Polyosteotic fibrous dysplasia, 9.7, 9.8, (90)

Popliteal cyst   6.13, (58)
Prepatellar bursitis   6.10, (58)
    infected   6.11, (58)
Pseudoarthrosis
    femoral shaft   5.11, (49)
    radius/ulna   2.4, 2.5, (16)
    tibia   9.5, (90)
Psoriasis   3.30, (35)

Radial nerve palsy   2.3, (16)
Radius
    distal fracture   3.14, (34)
    pseudoarthrosis   2.4, 2.5, (16)
Railing fracture   8.37, 8.38, 8.39, (84)
Rheumatoid arthritis   1.19, 1.23, (11), 9.3, (90)
    foot   8.20, 8.21, (84)
    hands   3.32, 3.33, 3.34, 3.35, (36)
    knee   6.7, (58), 9.3, (90)
    nodules   2.8, (16), 3.31, (36)
Rib hump   4.4, (43)
Rotator cuff rupture   1.16, 1.24, (11)

Sarcoma, soft tissue,   5.9, (49)
Scapula
    fixed   1.10, (11)
    winging   1.12, 1.13, 1.14, (11)
Scoliosis   4.4, (43), 9.6, (90)
Septic arthritis   1.15, (11), 5.1, (49)
Shoulder, Sprengel's   1.10, (11)
Shoulder dislocation   1.1, 1.2, 1.3, (11)
    habitual   1.4, 1.5, (11)
Simmond's test   8.41, (84)
Skin pigmentation   4.7, 4.8, (43), 9.7, (90)
Spina bifida
    aperta   4.9, 4.10, (43)
    occulta   4.6, (43)
Spinal infection/tumour   4.2, (43)
Spondylolisthesis   4.12, 4.13, (43)
Sprengel's shoulder   1.10, (11)
Sternoclavicular joint   1.15, (11)
Subacromial bursitis   1.19, (11)
Subdeltoid bursa   1.22, (11)
Subungual exostosis   8.33, 8.34, (84)
Subungual haematoma   3.22, (35)
Swan neck deformity   3.35, (36)
Syndactyly   3.4, (34)

Talipes equinavarus   8.1, 8.2, (83)
Talus, vertical   8.5, 8.6, (83)
Tenosynovitis
    acute suppurative   3.1, (34)
    de Quervain's   3.13, (34)
Thenar eminence, wasting   3.29, (35)
Thomas splint   5.2, (49)
Thomas's hip flexion   5.8, (49)
Thompson's test   8.41, (84)
Thumb
    forearm index   2.6, (16), 8.11, (83)
    Gamekeeper's   3.16, 3.17, 3.18, (34–35)
    mallet   3.19, (35)
    trigger   3.12, (34)
    ulnar collateral ligament rupture   3.16, 3.17,
        3.18, (34–35)
Tibia
    fracture   7.5, 7.8, (64)
    growth plate injury   8.37, 8.38, 8.39, (84)
    pseudoarthrosis   9.5, (90)
    vara (Blount's disease)   7.1, (64)
Tibialis posterior tendon rupture   8.40, (84)
Tibiofibular joint dislocation   6.12, (58)
Toe deformities   8.14, (83) See also specific
        deformities
Toenail
    deformity   8.32, (84)
    ingrowing   8.31, (84)
    subungual exostosis   8.33, 8.34, (84)
Toes, overriding   8.8, (83)
Torticollis   4.1, (43)

Ulna, pseudoarthrosis   2.4, 2.5, (16)
Ulnar drift   3.34, (36)
Ulnar nerve function test   3.26, 3.35, (35)
Ulnar nerve lesions   3.23, 3.24, 3.27, 3.28, (35)

Verruca   8.19, (83)
Vertical talus   8.5, 8.6, (83)
Volkmann's ischaemic contracture   2.2, (16), 8.29,
        8.30, (84)

Wrist
    drop   2.3, (16)
    synovitis   3.36, (36)
    trauma   3.15, (34)